*the* art *of*
wayfinding

# About the Author

Yoga and personal development teacher Meadow DeVor leads dozens of retreats, workshops, and training programs annually. She has worked in partnership with Wanderlust, Lululemon, and Recovery 2.0. Her writing has appeared at *Woman's Day*, *Elephant Journal*, YOGANONYMOUS, Teach.yoga, and the Good Men Project, and she has appeared on the *Oprah Winfrey Show*. You can listen to her weekly podcast and read more of her work on her website at www.MeadowDeVor.com. She lives with her family in a quiet beach town on California's Central Coast.

# Acknowledgments

Nothing is ever created by one person alone. I would like to express my gratitude not only to the people who helped bring this work into written form, but also to the people who helped me navigate the early terrain that brought me to this particular Point B.

To Martha Beck, my teacher, mentor, and friend: thank you for teaching me how to find my way home. To the Rowdies: this work wouldn't have come to light without your participation, self-study, and relentless inquiry. A special thanks to Ro Coury, for believing in this work, and for all her support and guidance in the first few years of helping me bring it into the world. Thank you to Kiley Schottenfeld, who was my right hand, a smiling face, and a constant source of support. To Lynn Swanson: if there are angels sent to help heal wounded souls, you are mine.

Thank you to Rebecca Gradinger, for your patience and your guidance. Thank you to Caroline Hemphill, for being equal parts editor, writing coach, and cheerleader. Thank you to Kent Dobson, who helped guide me through the daunting task of writing about the soul when mine had gone dark. Thank you to Laura McKowen for not only being my friend, but also for going through this entire first book publishing process right alongside me. There is a different kind of bond that forms in the trenches—I will be forever grateful that I shared the newbie author trench with you.

To Isabelle: you inspire me and make me want to be a better person. Thank you for breaking my heart wide open so that I could finally experience love.

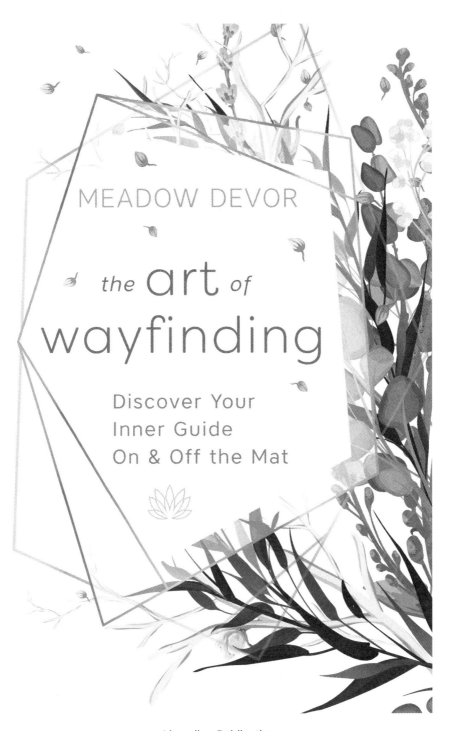

MEADOW DEVOR

the art of
wayfinding

Discover Your
Inner Guide
On & Off the Mat

Llewellyn Publications
Woodbury, Minnesota

FIRST EDITION
First Printing, 2020

Cover design by Kevin R. Brown
Editing by Rosemary Wallner
Interior yoga poses by the Llewellyn Art Department

Llewellyn Publications is a registered trademark of Llewellyn Worldwide Ltd.

Library of Congress Cataloging-in-Publication Data
Names: DeVor, Meadow, author.
Title: The art of wayfinding : discover your inner guide on & off the mat /
    Meadow DeVor.
Description: First edition. | Woodbury, Minnesota : Llewellyn Publications,
    2020. | Includes bibliographical references.
Identifiers: LCCN 2019039512 (print) | LCCN 2019039513 (ebook) | ISBN
    9780738760810 | ISBN 9780738761466 (ebook)
Subjects: LCSH: Yoga. | Meditation. | Contemplation. | Spirituality. |
    Self-actualization (Psychology)
Classification: LCC B132.Y6 D477 2020  (print) | LCC B132.Y6  (ebook) | DDC
    158.1—dc23
LC record available at https://lccn.loc.gov/2019039512
LC ebook record available at https://lccn.loc.gov/2019039513

Llewellyn Publications
A Division of Llewellyn Worldwide Ltd.
2143 Wooddale Drive
Woodbury, MN 55125-2989
www.llewellyn.com

Printed in the United States of America

## Other Books by Meadow DeVor

*Money Love (2011)*

*The Tao of Rowdy (2013)*

*For Lynn*
*—who never believed I was lost—*

# Contents

# Wayfinding Yoga Sequences

# Wayfinding Inquiry List

The art of wayfinding involves listening to each of your inner voices—Mind, Heart, Body, and Soul. Through the practice of inquiry, you can clarify the message of each voice, helping you understand the meaning, advice, or direction that the voice offers you. At the end of each section, you'll find an inquiry method designed to help you find your way with the guidance of that particular voice. At the end, you'll find an inquiry method that combines all four voices, helping you navigate with your whole self.

# The Practices: On the Mat and Off

# Disclaimer

The author offers the yoga postures and inquiry guides in this book as useful tools and advice for those who wish to transform their lives. The author has chosen not to include yoga pose scripts, and assumes that the reader either knows the pose or can easily look up how to do the pose. This book isn't intended to help the reader with the technical aspects of yoga poses. Rather, its intention is to help the reader use yoga to embody the tools within.

While the basic yoga postures in this book are intended to be gentle, readers should be aware of their own comfort level and know their limits. Before beginning a yoga practice, readers may want to consult their physician. This book is not intended as a substitute for the medical advice of physicians, and readers should always consult a physician in matters related to their health, and particularly with respect to any symptoms that may require diagnosis or medical attention.

In order to protect the privacy of individuals, the author may have changed the names of persons, places, or identifying characteristics and details of events and relationships.

"There is an Indian proverb or axiom that says that everyone is a house with four rooms, a physical, a mental, an emotional and a spiritual. Most of us tend to live in one room most of the time but, unless we go into every room every day, even if only to keep it aired, we are not a complete person."

*~Rumer Godden[1]*

1. Rumer Godden, *A House with Four Rooms* (New York: William Morrow & Company, 1989), 13.

# Introduction

In the middle of my life, I came to a crossroads and I didn't know which road to pick. It was as if I'd been snapped awake right there in the middle of the story, and I was lost.

I'm not the first person to land there. This freefall feeling of being adrift has been documented all the way back to the twelfth dynasty of Egypt. Dante, Aristotle, and essentially every poet, mystic, and hero since has spoken of it. Inevitably—whether it's Dorothy Gale, Luke Skywalker, Harry Potter, or you—there comes a point when you have to navigate through tough terrain without clear landmarks or any view of the horizon. You'll reach a point where all your old maps and compasses no longer work.

Maybe this is exactly where you find yourself right now. Maybe you feel like you're living in a shell, overwhelmed, lost, or alone. Maybe you've worked all your life, nose down and diligent, only to end up in a place you don't love, in a life that doesn't feel like your own. Or maybe you just have a sense that something is missing even if you don't exactly know what you're looking for.

Since time began, people have had to learn various navigation skills to help them find their way through this unknown and sometimes scary territory. Some learned to chart their course by starlight, some by listening to birdsong, others through reading faint water patterns off the bows of their boats. No matter the culture or method of travel, people have continuously turned to the art of wayfinding to find their answers and their way through to inner peace and understanding. Wayfinding is a skill to be mastered and requires focus, sharp listening, and an eye for subtle clues.

Journeying through life requires similar skills. Even if you don't know where you are or which direction you're going, you can learn how to live as your whole self. You have a built-in navigation system, a failproof tool to help you steer your life. You're probably already aware of your inner voice, and maybe you already use it.

But, the question is: Which inner voice are you listening to?

There's the Mind Voice who's trying to make everything predictable and safe. There's the Heart Voice who's relaying directions through a vast range of emotions. There's the Body Voice who's driven by animal instincts. And then there's the Soul Voice who propels you to live the fullest expression of who you are. Each voice holds its own sense of direction, a unique piece of the puzzle, and its own corner of the map. When used together, the Four Voices become a powerful inner guidance system.

Through inquiry and yoga, I'll show you how each inner voice has a distinctly different communication style and wildly divergent motives, and how each offers contradictory feedback that can be really confusing to navigate. As you fine-tune your inner-listening skills, you'll not only learn to steer your life using the wisdom of each of the Four Voices, but you'll also find a way to deepen your connection to loved ones, to who you really are, and to life itself.

In the "on the mat" section of each chapter, you'll embody wayfinding techniques through inquiry within your yoga practice. These practices will help you to deepen your understanding of each inner voice, beyond just reading words on a page. In the "off the mat" portion of each chapter, I'll relate what you've experienced "on the mat" to the larger life lessons, showing you how to take that particular aspect of your yoga and inquiry practice out into the world.

## My Story

My career in yoga and self-development began over twenty years ago, but it wasn't until I had the privilege of working with a remarkable group of women for nearly a decade that I began to develop the powerful tools you'll find within this book.

Each week, I taught my students—first via teleconference, eventually via video conference—a new tool, a new concept, or a new practice. Pulling from philosophy, poetry, psychology, neuroscience, spiritual texts, and mythology, my weekly classes focused on a myriad of self-development topics. Whether the focus was on deepening a sense of purpose, strengthening boundaries, building stronger relationships, or healing one's relationship to money, the topics always had one thing in common: how to find your way through a human life. As part of this ongoing class, I also facilitated a private forum where my students could share their class work, disclose current challenges, and receive help from me and one another.

While most of my colleagues worked with small groups for a few weeks at a time, I studied the innermost thoughts and feelings of over a hundred women, from five different continents, over the span of nine and a half years. This unique opportunity gave me an unprecedented viewpoint. From this perspective, I witnessed what worked well—meaning what tools and techniques helped my students achieve what they desired—and more importantly, I learned which tools didn't stand up to the test of time.

In 2014, I came to a crossroads. The night before my winter break began, I opened my laptop, hoping to jot down a few sentences to let my students know that I'd be offline for a few days. When I opened my account, however, I found a staggering number of emails; my students were in the throes of the special set of challenges that the holidays offer: travel and holiday expenses, stress from having their families under the same roof, overwhelm from a ten-mile-long to-do list, anxiety from lack of routine—all common issues for that time of year.

Other students were spiraling around the same struggles that they had been battling again and again: drinking problems, bingeing, chronic loneliness, depression, and unresolved issues from their childhood. These were smart women, successful women—Harvard and Stanford grads, lawyers, doctors, prosperous business owners, and accomplished athletes—women who read and studied, actively applying the tools they had learned. These women were some of my star students, women who had diligently done their work. Yet, no matter how much work they had done, they still seemed to carry the same old stress and anxiety, the same addictions and compulsions, the same cycle of suffering.

For years, I had opened my laptop and replied to my students' posts, hoping to leave them feeling a little bit better, offering them some clarity, truth, and understanding. But that night, I just couldn't make myself do it. I didn't type a single word because I'd already said everything that I knew to say. I had no new tools, I had no new perspectives. I didn't know why some of the women permanently changed their lives while others couldn't. I couldn't figure out why some seemed to evolve while others stayed stuck. I was exasperated, confused, and discouraged. My heart ached for my students. I didn't want to surrender my belief that there was a way to break through their patterns of suffering and I didn't want to close up shop. Yet, I felt like I'd come to a place where I either had to walk away and admit defeat, or I had to find a better method for teaching.

I spent that winter break feeling lost, confused, and beat down. Yet, beneath that, the love of my work, my devotion to my students, and the undying curiosity beneath my discouragement propelled me forward. By the end of the holiday, I decided there had to be something I'd missed. There had to be a reason for the disparity within my group. And I was determined to find it.

Over the next few months, I relentlessly read everything I could find on the long-term effects of trauma, dove deeper into studying the mysteries of addiction, and began combing through my student body, looking for patterns that might help me find answers. One book in particular, written by the founder and medical director of the Trauma Center in Brookline, Massachusetts, spoke directly to me. In *The Body Keeps the Score*, Dr. Bessel Van Der Kolk showed how trauma literally reshapes both body and brain, compromising one's capacity for pleasure, engagement, self-control, and trust. He said traumatized people often keep repeating the same problems and have trouble learning from their experience. He spoke of the shortcomings of traditional treatments and explored several innovative treatments in the book—from neurofeedback and meditation to sports, drama, equine therapy, and yoga—as these activities allow the body to have experiences that contradict the helplessness of trauma.[2]

Informed with this perspective, I sifted through thousands of forum posts, class discussions, and private emails. I made notes about individual traumas and addictions. I asked my students to share what else they were doing outside of the group and made a list of physical and spiritual practices that they'd found to be an integral part of their growth.

An unexpected pattern emerged.

Most of my students were quite adept at the mind-based inquiry methods that I share in this book. Within that group, a smaller number had basic tools for understanding and allowing natural-flowing emotion. But I found that the women who had made the biggest transformations also had personal practices that involved their physical bodies as well as having a spiritual practice. These women did yoga, or they loved to run. They had a weekly dance class, or they worked with horses. In addition, they were active in their church, or they felt deeply connected to nature. They had personal practices of prayer, contemplation, and meditation, or they believed in a higher purpose for themselves.

After months of research, I had a hunch. Online, I'd been solely teaching variations of cognitive tools—what I now call the Mind Voice—primarily focusing on the logical reasoning skills of the mind. I'd barely scratched the surface of the vast realm of emotion—the heart—and had completely skipped the body and the soul. Yet, when I led retreats, I always included a physical component—whether it was horse whispering, yoga classes, hiking, or ropes courses. And I also included a soul component—meditation, mantras, labyrinth walking, or prayer. Students came away from those weekend retreats radically transformed. Those experiences seemed to have exponentially stronger potency than my online classes. I had always chalked these differences up to the power of the group, or to the beauty of the location. But after combing through thousands of pages of information, I wondered if the real difference came down to teaching to all four parts of a person: Mind, Heart, Body, and Soul.

---

2. Bessel A Van der Kolk, *The Body Keeps the Score: Brain, Mind, and Body in the Healing of Trauma* (New York: Viking, 2014), 3, 150–151, 213, 263–276.

In my personal life, I'd always seen my yoga mat as a place to intentionally practice self-development tools. On the yoga mat, I not only practiced stilling the voice of my mind, but I also opened my heart to the experience of my emotions, brought awareness to the subtleties of my physical body, and discovered a profound depth of spirituality. Through this practice of connection and intentional conversation with my inner voices, I'd leave the mat with a clear sense of inner guidance.

If I wanted to help my students create deeply meaningful lives, I needed to help them reliably access all four parts of themselves with or without being on retreat. I needed to teach them how to go beyond the voice of the mind. I needed to teach them to listen to the voice of their heart, the voice of their body, and the voice of their soul. Through the integration of the Four Voices, I believed my students could learn to find their way and rely on their own sense of inner guidance.

I first taught the Four Voices to my women's group and saw immediate and remarkable changes. When the women addressed all Four Voices, issues that typically took weeks to work through in conversation suddenly surfaced within minutes. Women who previously wouldn't leave toxic situations began to set healthy boundaries. Women who'd always hated their bodies found a depth of love and appreciation for their own skin. Women who'd always lived in financial fear found a sense of inner security and trust. By using the inner guidance of all Four Voices, students began to feel safe and strong enough to live as the fullest expression of who they were always meant to be.

Since then, I've taught thousands of men and women to use their Four Voices as an inner guidance system—on and off the yoga mat. I incorporated all Four Voices into my trainings, workshops, classes, and retreats. Online and in person, I've shown my students how to embody these techniques while on the yoga mat—similar to the "on the mat" practices within this book.

I have spent decades developing and testing techniques and practices from the fields of self-development, psychology, spirituality, philosophy, and yoga. Through my research and through my own personal experience,

I've distilled and refined this list down to the tried-and-true wayfinding essentials that I share in this book.

Whether you find yourself at a crossroads, a little lost, or completely stuck, working with the Four Voices will help you through the confusion. You'll no longer feel torn and conflicted, and you'll begin to move through life with deliberate clarity. Rather than living up in your head, you'll find you are a complex and beautiful human being with a vast array of emotions, with animal instincts refined over eons, and with a soul that continually wants you to expand and grow. By staying in conversation with all Four Voices, you'll discover the art of wayfinding—your innate ability to chart your course and find your way home.

As you start to listen to the Four Voices and to navigate using the wisdom of your whole self, you'll discover a renewed source of inspiration and strength. No longer lost, you'll find yourself standing firmly on solid ground. Inspired and transformed, your sense of direction will be sharpened, and the path forward will become clear. Let this book serve as a compass to help you find your way.

chapter one

# How It Works

If you take a look at your life as it is right now, you'll see a complex land-scape of things you do well and things that maybe you don't do so well. Maybe you're really organized in one part of your life but there's a lot of chaos in another. Maybe you're disciplined and motivated when it comes to taking care of your body but you lack a sense of deep intimacy and find yourself feeling lonely. Or maybe you're entirely lost and have no idea who you are, what you want, or where to start. Wherever you currently find yourself, whether your life might need some slight tweaks or a complete overhaul, imagine this specific place of your life being marked on a map. Imagine that where you are right now is stamped with a big red X in the middle of the map of your life. Let's call this Point A.

Now let's say you want to change something. You don't want to be at Point A anymore. Something is not quite right about this place in your life. Maybe you want to have more meaningful relationships. Maybe you want to excel in your profession. Maybe you've never finished anything in your life, and so are determined to finish the scarf you started to knit two win-ters ago. Whether your change is tiny or daunting, there's somewhere you want to go. Even if you're lost, even if you don't really know where you want to go, what you want to change, or how to do it—you know there's a place out there you're trying to get to. Let's call your desired destination Point B.

To get to Point B, you have to take a journey and there are countless ways to do this. You can meander and spiral and go backward and forward.

You can go slow or fast. You can take the scenic route or the expressway. No matter how you do it, if you have a reliable navigation system or even a good sense of direction, you'll eventually get to Point B.

But if you're not paying attention, if you're distracted, checked out, or sleepwalking through your life—it's impossible to orient yourself. Landmarks are missed because you're not paying attention. Your navigation system fails because you're not listening. Your sense of direction is confusing and unreliable. You have no idea whether you're supposed to go left or go right. You have no way of knowing if you're getting closer to Point B or farther away. You may never get there. You are completely lost with no compass to guide you.

For example, let's say your Point B is to finish knitting a scarf. To get to this destination, you have several things you must do. You must buy yarn and knitting needles. You must learn basic knitting stitches. And then you must knit each stitch of each row until it's complete. This doesn't have to happen all in one sitting; but over time, if you continue to stitch rows, you will end up at Point B: a completed scarf.

But sometimes it's not quite that easy. Sometimes you have every intention of getting to Point B but somewhere along the way you get distracted. Let's say you buy yarn and knitting needles and you learn the basic knitting stitches. But then you stitch one row and decide that it doesn't look right it, so you unravel your work and start over. And then you try it again and decide it isn't right, so you unravel it again and start over. And then you get frustrated and bored, so you get up off the couch and go see if you have any good snacks. You find a bag of pretzels and bring them back to the couch. You look at the knitting, but it's hard to knit when you have food in your hands, so you turn on the TV instead. You watch an episode of *Grey's Anatomy* and—let's be honest—it's impossible not to watch the next one because: cliffhanger. You watch one more episode promising yourself you'll get back to your knitting. Three hours later, you've finished season six, eaten the entire bag of pretzels, and you're sitting next to a heap of tangled yarn.

The first example gets you to Point B: the finished scarf. The second example, where you got distracted, took you to a different destination: not

Point B. Nothing about this is rocket science; it's actually pretty simple and easy to understand how one person ends up with a knitted scarf when another ends up with an empty pretzel bag and a fistful of yarn. The difficult part is understanding why. Why does one person end up with the knitted scarf? Why did that person continue to stitch row after row? How did that person end up with the discipline to learn, to keep going, to finish? And why does another person have all the best intentions of finishing, but instead gets distracted and never finishes?

Maybe you don't care about knitting a scarf. Maybe you want to stop drinking, run a marathon, or launch a new business. Maybe you don't even know what you want to do, you just know you don't want this. This life that you're sitting in. This mess. This loneliness. This frustration.

This is the crux of my work as a coach and a teacher, what the tools in this book are and what I've devoted most of my professional life to—teaching wayfinding skills that get you to Point B. As you learn more about the Four Voices and how to use them, you'll use your inner guidance system to steer your life in the right direction. It won't always be a direct route to your destination, and you may get lost again, but you can learn how to rely on these tools to locate your true self whenever you are off track, and to help you get from a thousand Point As to a thousand Point Bs.

But first, we need to know who's driving your car.

## Who's Driving?

Imagine a car. Make it whatever style you like, as long as it's small, doesn't have all the modern bells and whistles, and only seats five people. Now imagine you have four passengers in the car.

The first passenger is Soul. She's sitting shotgun and holding a compass. It's a special compass, not really a north, south, east, west type of thing. Soul's compass is rigged to point in one direction—for now, let's just call the direction *warmer*. This doesn't necessarily tell you how to get somewhere. Sometimes Soul takes you right up to a brick wall or to a dead-end road. Sometimes the bridge goes out and you're just sitting at the edge of a huge crevasse. Sometimes *warmer* means not going anywhere at all.

Soul's compass holds critical wisdom, which we'll get to later in the book. To start with, just know that Soul isn't very clear about whether you're supposed to take a left on 15th Street or a right on Sunset Boulevard. She's not bothered by the details of the journey such as roadblocks and washed-out bridges; she just sits quietly with her compass and whispers obscure directions from time to time. She sees the journey from a much higher perspective, knowing that if you keep moving toward *warmer*, you'll eventually get where you want to go.

Soul dreams bigger than your biggest imagination: she wants more for you than you have ever dared to dream so finding a way to trust this wise voice is essential. But trusting this voice may feel awkward and impractical at first, especially when you're a human and live on the ground. To get where you want to go, you need to be able to navigate yourself through streets and over bridges. You need to find the mountain pass and know where to cross the rivers. You need to know how to get yourself safely through the deserts and how to avoid the swamps. You need to chart a route down to the smallest detail. You need to recognize milestones, landmarks, and signs as you pass them. You need to change course if you make a wrong turn. For specific navigation like this, you need more than just your compass, you also need a map.

That's where your other passengers come in.

In the backseat are three other passengers: Mind, Heart, and Body. Did you picture them as adults? If so, change them to kids. Your kids. I like to think of Mind, Heart, and Body as children because it's a lot easier to have compassion and understanding for little kids. Plus, as you'll learn throughout this book, these kids often misbehave. So, I'd much rather you picture a tantrum coming from a cute little toddler instead of a grumpy old man.

Your kids hold the map. To be more precise, each kid has one-third of the map. Each portion of the map is critical but incomplete. To successfully navigate, you need all three pieces of the map. When the kids in the backseat get along, they work together and you have a reliable map. You're able to count on Soul for the compass and the kids for the detailed minute-by-minute navigation. Through the countryside, cityscapes, and scenic routes, everyone works together to get you to Point B. Of course, if you've ever driven anywhere with three kids in the back of a small car, you know that this sort of peace and harmony doesn't last for long.

Before you know it, Mind wants to be in charge. She's very noisy and talks incessantly. It's like having a little commentator in the backseat who never shuts up. She tells you if she hates your driving, or if she likes your driving (which is almost never). She wants you to stop, she wants you to go left, she wants you to hurry, she wants you to slow down. You can never really make her happy. Whatever you're doing, she'll find something that could be better, something that should be different. She thinks her map is the only true map and constantly tries to talk over her siblings when they offer help.

Then Heart takes over. She's very emotional and feels everything deeply. She can be all swoony and in love one minute, then vile and hateful in the next. And when she's sad, she's really sad. When she's mad, she's really mad. From terror, to joy, to shame, to calm—she is a rainbow of emotion. She doesn't have to say much; her mood affects the entire car.

Body sits silently in the backseat taking notes in her diary. She's a little more introverted and not as talkative as her siblings. Often, she gets completely overlooked. She doesn't interrupt and patiently waits for her turn. She goes along for the ride and she's a pretty good sport most of the time. But every so often Body gets fed up. Eventually, she gets sick of being ignored and frustrated when her map isn't taken seriously. At which point, she ever-so-graciously pulls the emergency brake, bringing the entire car to a screeching halt. Until she's happy, no one goes anywhere.

Whether the kids are in agreement or offering confusing and contradictory directions, you're the one in the driver's seat. The more present and connected you are, the easier it is to listen to each of the Four Voices. The better you are at understanding each of the voices in the car, which part of the map they hold, and the specific gifts and weaknesses of each voice, the better you are at charting your course.

This is what it looks like to live from a state of connection. When you're connected—or in a state of conscious awareness—you're in the driver's seat.

You're able to communicate and listen to feedback from all Four Voices. You know that each of your kids has valuable information to share and you take each of their ideas into consideration. Even if the kids are fighting, you're able to reason with them and work it out. You're able to have an open line of conversation with Soul and you work together to figure out where you want to go. You're aware of your surroundings. You're moving toward your desired destination. Life is good.

Now let's say you've had a bad day at work and you just can't take one more thing. You've had it up to here with life, your boss, and your stupid coworker who always takes the last of the coffee. You're distracted and tired and you just want to check out.

So you crawl into the backseat of your imaginary car and take a nap. Soul stays in the passenger's seat and kids one, two, and three take the driver's seat. Just take a moment to picture this. Remember, this is a tiny car, so you're curled up and not very comfortable in the back. The driver's seat doesn't offer a lot of room and now you have three kids jockeying for the wheel. I might be stating the obvious, but this is not ideal.

While you're checked out in the backseat, chaos takes over. The kids drive and no one watches them. Soul tries to wake you up with her whispers but you can't hear her because there's too much noise. Mind takes the wheel while Heart and Body try to wrestle her little hands away. Heart takes over and Mind starts screaming at the top of her lungs. Body keeps trying to hit the brakes. The car is out of control. Mayhem ensues. They drive around in circles, they hit objects along the way, they get lost and have no idea where they are.

Eventually, you wake up and take a look at the wreckage around you. Sometimes that wreckage looks like an empty pretzel bag and a tangled mess of yarn. This is what happens when you are distracted, disconnected, and sleepwalking through life. The kids take the wheel.

This is why you ended up on the couch with the clicker instead of putting on your walking shoes after work and walking your three miles. This is why you ended up spending $416 at Target when you only went in for shampoo. This is why your mother-in-law is coming to stay with you for six weeks when you promised yourself you'd never be in the same room with her again. The kids are at the wheel.

This is why you feel lost—you went to sleep in the backseat and forgot that you're supposed to be the driver of your life.

It's time to wake up.

## How to Stay Awake

This book is about waking up and staying awake. It's about being present and connected so you can stay in the driver's seat and navigate to Point B. If you sleepwalk through your life, you will have to learn to practice waking up fully in your life and remaining fully present, and yoga is the best method I've found for learning this. When I can teach you to stay awake on your mat, you can translate these lessons into the rest of your life. Think of the practice of yoga as going deeper and deeper into a state of connection and awareness. As you become more aware, you're able to work with the Four Voices, integrating their messages to create change with awareness and ease. If you fall back into old patterns and lose touch with the Four Voices, you risk losing your natural sense of direction. You then become more easily distracted and reactive and are therefore less capable of navigating difficult terrain, or creating lasting change.

## On the Mat: Get in the Driver's Seat

### *Lie on the Mat*

Lie on your back and close your eyes. The easiest way to deepen your connection—to be fully here—is through your senses.

Slow your breath down, close your mouth, and inhale deeply through your nose. Feel the quality of the air as it comes in through your nostrils. Exhale through your nose. Feel the quality of the air as it exits through your nostrils. Maybe the air is warmer as you exhale and cooler as you inhale. Just notice what it feels like to breathe through your nose. Practice lengthening your breath: count to four as you inhale and then count to four as you exhale.

Continue your breath. Feel your body sink into the floor. The weight of your feet, your thighs, your hips, your shoulders as you release your entire body into the floor. Feel all the points on your body where you are being held and supported by the floor.

Listen to your surroundings. Maybe you hear a car alarm off in the distance, or a plane flying overhead. Maybe you hear the neighbor's dog barking, or the hum of your refrigerator. Can you still hear your breath as you inhale and exhale? What else do you hear? How far away are the sounds? Are they soft or loud? Can you just observe the sounds around you and then let them go?

Notice any aromas in the air. Maybe you smell your laundry detergent on your clothes, or the incense you lit before your practice. What do you smell? Can you observe the scents around you and then let them go?

Notice the taste in your mouth. Maybe you just brushed your teeth and you still taste the minty residue. Maybe you just finished a cup of coffee and can taste the lingering mellow earthiness. What do you taste? Can you observe the taste and then let it go?

Keeping your gaze relaxed, open your eyes and slowly observe your surroundings. Maybe you see a candle flickering, an empty journal in front of you, or a copy of this book. What do you see? Can you allow yourself to see your surroundings without getting involved with them? Can you just observe them and then let them go?

Can you still hear your breath as you inhale and exhale? Can you still feel the air as it rushes through your throat, making soft ocean sounds?

This practice of presence brings you into full awareness of each of your senses. Sensory information is available to you all the time. At any point in your practice, you can tune in to any or all of your five senses. You can return to conscious breath, listening to the ocean-like sounds of your inhale and your exhale. This is the practice of yoga, of connection. Take a moment to really experience what it feels like to be here now. This is what it feels like to be in the driver's seat. You're here. You're connected to this moment. You're awake.

Breathe.

Now, I'm going to have you move to the backseat of your car. Don't worry, I'll bring you right back to the front seat, but I want you to experience both connection and distraction. What it's like to be the driver and what it's like to be checked out in the backseat while you're on your mat. The easiest way to do this is to think about something that's worrying you. Something unfinished. Something that's nagging at you. Take a moment to find your topic.

What happened when you did this? What did that feel like?

To think about the future or to worry about your problems, you have to stop being present with here and now. You probably stopped feeling your body on the mat. Maybe you stopped noticing the birds singing outside. Maybe you stopped noticing the scent of your burning candle. And I'm guessing your breathing quickened and became more erratic. At the very least, I bet you stopped listening to your breath because you stopped being here to witness it. You severed the connection with this moment. That's what disconnection feels like. That's what it feels like to check out and move to the backseat. It's like part of you is still on the mat and part of you went off to think about the future or the past. Your body is still in the pose, but the kids are driving the car now.

I'll be honest: I used to go to yoga to do exactly this. I thought it was the perfect place to go to think. I actually thought it was designed *for* thinking. I would get on my mat and bring all my problems and irritations with me and then I'd sort through them one by one while I sorta-kinda listened to the teacher. I was off planning Friday's dinner party or writing that email that had to be sent. I was busy working through grievances or entertaining myself with fantasies. Preoccupied and distracted, my body would somehow go through the poses. But you know what ended up happening? I kept getting hurt. I kept over-stretching and I'd leave my yoga class feeling worse off than when I'd arrived. I didn't know how to stay in the driver's seat. I didn't even know that I should try to stay in the driver's seat. The minute I got on the mat, I hopped in the backseat and went on autopilot while the kids drove the car.

In yoga, the goal isn't to just move your body through shapes and poses and then to lie down at the end of class. I mean, maybe that's helpful for some people, but that's not the depth and meaning behind the practice. The practice isn't really about the pose, it's not about whether or not you balanced on your left foot for all five breaths, or if you can do a perfect handstand. It's actually quite possible to do those things and more, even when you're in the backseat planning your next vacation. The more meaningful practice of yoga is about connecting to yourself. It's about staying awake so you can listen to all Four Voices. It's about whether you can stay here, now, on your mat. From this space, we can take the practice even deeper and begin listening to the Four Voices.

## Off the Mat: Get in the Driver's Seat

Whether you're sitting in your dentist's office, waiting in your car for your kids to get out of school, or cooking dinner for your family, being awake—staying in the driver's seat—takes practice.

So let's imagine you just arrived at your dentist's office. You come into the office, check in at the desk, and turn around to find a seat to wait your turn. And then, what do you do?

I'm guessing you pull out your phone.

This is where I want you to stop. Because this is a moment where it's really easy to jump in the backseat, check out, and go to sleep. It's easy to open your phone. It's easy to scroll through your texts. It's easy to click on Instagram, check your email, or play a game. Even if you just pull it out for a quick minute, scroll through your different notifications and put the phone right back in your pocket—it's almost impossible to do this from the driver's seat. Why? Think about what else you could do if you didn't. You'd quietly sit in a room with other humans. You might even have to look them in the eye. You might even feel the need to strike up a conversation with them. Or you might feel a sense of unpleasant restlessness as you sit in the silence. This is not easy. It's uncomfortable. To avoid this discomfort, you climb into the backseat, grab your phone, and entertain yourself.

But our goal is to stay in the driver's seat, to practice staying awake. So, instead of your habitual grab-my-phone response, practice the same tool you learned on your mat.

While you sit in the waiting room, pick a place in the room to focus on. Bring your eyes to a soft gaze. Close your mouth and inhale deeply through your nose. Feel your body sink into your chair. Feel your feet on the ground. Listen to your surroundings. Simply observe the sounds around you and then let them go. Notice any aromas in the air. Without becoming involved with them, simply notice them and let them go. Become aware of the taste in your mouth. Simply observe the taste and then let it go. Keeping your gaze relaxed, observe your surroundings. Allow yourself to look at your surroundings without getting involved with them. Just observe them and then let them go.

No matter where you find yourself, you can use this practice of presence to bring yourself into the driver's seat. You can tune in to any or all of your five senses. You can return to the practice of conscious breath. This is the practice of yoga off the mat. This is the practice of being connected. No matter where you are, take a moment to really experience what it feels like to be here now. This is what it feels like to be in the driver's seat. You're here. You're connected to this moment. You're awake.

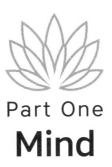

## Part One
# Mind

From criticisms to judgments, future worries, or re-enacting scenarios from the past, the Mind Voice often clutters your perception, confusing you and making it difficult to navigate the present. In this section, you'll learn how to recognize the Mind Voice and how it functions.

Once you can easily identify the Mind Voice, I'll show you how to use this voice for navigation—giving you a detailed overview of Mind's portion of the map—and show you how to use it while you're in the driver's seat. Next, I'll show you what happens when you're asleep in the backseat and your anxious mind starts wildly steering the car. To conclude this section, I'll share a tool to help you deepen your connection to the Mind Voice so you can fine-tune your inner navigation system. As we move through each of these chapters, I'll walk you through an experience on the mat to help you embody these tools and then we'll take the practice off the mat and into real life.

# chapter two

# The Mind Voice

An introduction to the voice of the mind.
How it works, how to recognize it,
and how it influences your journey.

I live with an inner nag, an anxious busybody who never shuts up. From the minute I wake up to the minute I go to sleep, I can hear her blabbing on and on about everything she sees and every tiny thing that is wrong with me and the world. Most of us were never trained in how to deal with this voice. Instead, we just put up with the endless stream of insults, judgments, and fears. My inner bitch has got a bullhorn up to my brain. Her voice is persistent and unrelenting. There's no escaping her.

As I type this, I can hear her in the background, yarning on.

"I'm never going to be able to finish this chapter. I'm not a writer. Who do I think I am? What should I make for dinner? God, I'm sick of salad. Why can't I just have potato chips? I need to be healthy. I should go vegan. Did I forget to change over the laundry? I think Kristin is mad; I should probably apologize. Screw Kristin! If she's mad, that's her own damned problem. I should check my email. I hate email."

At this point, I'm now just staring at a blank screen with a blinking cursor. No creativity happens when I am listening to this voice in my head. She's a maniac who contradicts herself constantly and treats me terribly.

This inner commentator is the Mind Voice. Maybe yours is kinder and gentler, but I doubt it. Maybe yours is ultra-efficient, yelling out to-do lists

24/7. Maybe yours is going on and on about how the neighbor's dog needs to stop barking, or maybe your inner voice is insecure and keeps you up all night, tossing and turning, wondering if that dude is ever going to call.

Who would you be without that voice in your head? Calmer? Happier? Would you be more confident? More productive?

## The Inner Commentator

Whether you go to your local yoga studio or an ashram in India, the practice begins the same way: you roll out your mat, find a comfortable position, and wait for class to begin. Everything that happened leading up to class, including traffic, weather, texts, emails, deadlines, and shopping lists, are put aside when you arrive at class. You come in, sit on your mat, and pause. This process of arriving requires you to slow down, settle into yourself and find a deliberate respite. Sometimes your mind races and it's hard to let go of what just happened before you got to class. Other times, it's easier to find a peaceful state, to calm yourself. This process—settling the mind before you even do the first pose or take the first inhale—is the first step in yoga.

The voice in your head follows you into class. She talks about what you're wearing and criticizes you or others around you. She talks about whether the check-in process was good or bad or whether or not Suzy behind the desk smiled at you in the right way. If you just stop and listen, you'll hear your Mind Voice opining about all sorts of details. It's too hot. It's too cold. The music is too loud. It's too quiet in here. And then your Mind Voice spots someone—you know—*that* person. And then the Mind Voice starts in with commentary about how they're prettier, smarter, skinnier, better, more popular, healthier, younger, more flexible. *Blah blah blah.*

This voice does not stop once you come to the top of the mat. This voice follows you through every inhale, every pose, every transition, and every exhale. This inner commentator ranks, judges, critiques, hassles, congratulates, and is all caught up in what other people are doing, what you look like, and what other people might be thinking of you. This voice has ideas about what the teacher should or shouldn't be doing, what the person next to you should or shouldn't be doing. This voice has a laundry list of changes that it would like to enforce to make this class, this experience, this pose fit some particular scripted version of the world. This voice, when it's running the show, is exhausting. And this voice is not you, it is merely the Mind Voice trying to make the world around you behave, to make it predictable so you can be safe.

## Who Is She and Why Does She Talk So Much?

To be fair, the inner commentator—or Mind Voice—is only one aspect of your vast, complex, and beautiful brain. So, let's get clear on what the Mind Voice actually is and what it's not. I am not a neuroscientist so I'll keep the anatomy lesson as basic and relevant as possible. I've found that a brief bit of science helps set the stage before we dive into the more obscure realms of the Mind Voice.

The Mind Voice comes from part of your brain. Although the terms "brain" and "mind" are often used interchangeably, for the purposes of our work, there's a slight difference between the two. For starters, you can see a brain. Your brain is an organ in your body, like your lungs, spleen, or kidneys. It is tangible. When I talk about the mind, I am referring to the intangible world of thoughts, ideas, perceptions, beliefs, and imagination.

Your brain keeps your heart beating, your lungs breathing, and helps to ensure you put your hands out to brace yourself if you fall. Your brain also houses a mind that can write symphonies and poems and love songs. Your mind can design skyscrapers and bridges and belt buckles. It can remind you to put a stamp on the envelope before you put it in the mailbox, and it can conjure up the memory of your grandma's kitchen. In this way, the mind can be creative, innovative, and inspiring. But, this isn't the part of the mind that I'm referring to in the Four Voices. For the purposes of this work, when I refer to the Mind Voice, I'm talking about the voice inside your head that's often critical, judgmental, envious, full of rage, or ready to bolt.

The Mind Voice comes from a tiny part of the brain called the amygdala. If you imagine drawing a line between your ears, and visualize two almonds positioned along that line, one behind each eye, you'd have a good idea of the general shape, size, location, and origin of this little beast of a voice. The almonds—amygdalae—are part of your limbic system. The limbic system, also known as the "reptilian brain" or the "emotional brain," takes in information through your senses and attaches an emotion to it.

The amygdala serves as the triage master for all incoming information. Information comes in through the senses and those little almonds go to work sorting and ranking the potential threats, determining whether you're safe or at risk. When things are familiar and predictable, your little almonds are nice and quiet. But life on planet Earth is never all that predictable—reality is a constant barrage of things that change, things that are unfamiliar, and things that put us at risk. These threats trigger the amygdala's fear/rage response, raising your brain's level of anxiety so you can pay attention and eliminate the threat.[3]

This is very helpful when you encounter something dangerous such as a brush fire, a rattlesnake, or when a mountain lion wanders into your suburban backyard while you are sipping a glass of iced tea on the patio. The problem is that this voice in your head is sometimes just as loud no matter what the worry is: whether it's a mountain lion or a bad hair day. To her, both are deemed dangerous. Both are triaged as threats. To her, everything is an emergency and everything (and everyone) needs to be controlled. Think of the Mind Voice as a software system designed to keep you safe. This primitive part of your brain was handed down from your ancestors and evolved to keep you fed, watered, warm, and away from predators. It also kept you safe from acts of nature or attacks from neighboring tribes. It kept you safe within your own tribe so you weren't exiled because that would have meant certain death.

Imagine all that history and all that beautiful programming that once kept humans safe from famine, flood, blizzards, and bear attacks, now being funneled into whether or not an Instagram post got enough likes, or whether your coworker is talking behind your back, or whether someone swiped right. Impending danger triggers a very old part of our brain, and when that part gets freaked out, that screaming worry won't stop its urgent nagging.

---

3. Jill Bolte Taylor, *My Stroke of Insight: A Brain Scientist's Personal Journey* (New York: Viking, 2008), 15–18.

## What Language Does She Speak?

Out of the Four Voices, you can easily spot the Mind Voice because she's the only one that sounds like a person in your head. Her language is words, thoughts, and beliefs. She speaks in sentences, questions, and sidebar commentary. She can mimic voices from your past—she might do a brilliant impression of your mother or your second-grade teacher or your ex-husband. She can grab pieces of past conversations—usually the things you wished you could forget—and embed them in your head like a Katy Perry song, replaying them over and over. Whether you're on the mat or off, she's your thinking voice, your ruminating voice, your scenario-imagining voice. If you're feeling anxious or bored, this is the voice that starts to tell you a story. Maybe it's a story about your past, something that happened to you years ago and the Mind Voice lulls you with an old familiar tale. Maybe it's a story about a possible future, and Mind Voice entertains you with all the possibilities. Maybe she's criticizing you or criticizing those around you. Maybe she's running possible scripts to use for a sticky situation.

Even though this voice might sound like your own voice, she's not you. The Mind Voice is merely a software system running strategies to control and predict possible threats. Her voice isn't personal. She isn't against you, trying to hurt your feelings or sabotage you. She's not really *for* you either. The Mind Voice is simply a ticker tape of thoughts, sentences, and conversation on an everlasting loop. Still, the Mind Voice carries an important piece of the puzzle, and if you can drop beyond the clutter, this voice can soften and inform.

## Journaling

One morning, a few poses into the community morning yoga class, I noticed that I was having a difficult time settling down. The teacher had started us off gently, bringing our attention to our seat and our breath—a typical start to a yoga class. But my mind kept jumping from one thing to the next. I wasn't stressed. I wasn't worried. My mind was just busy, it wanted to think-think-think. We moved to our backs in what was supposed to be a deep meditation. Stillness and quiet surrounded me as my classmates settled in. But my mind kept on running all over the place. I've practiced yoga for a long time, so I'm not too alarmed by the daily fluctuations. Sometimes my body is rickety and sometimes it isn't. Sometimes I'm emotional, sometimes I'm not. Sometimes my mind just wants to run around and be busy, making it more difficult to arrive on the mat and to be fully present.

This is just one of the many reasons I recommend that you keep a journal nearby while you practice yoga. Having a pen and paper is an important part of wayfinding work. First, it serves as a place to record insights. It also serves as a way to get clutter out of your mind. You might use your journal as a place to write down beautiful questions to ponder, as a place to scribble your grocery list, or as a space to mind dump all the negative self-talk, stressful thoughts, or the habitual worries that creep into your mind during class. By journaling these thoughts, you'll find that you are able to get them on paper and out of your mind for the time being.

The goal of creating stillness and quiet in yoga isn't to erase the self. It is to allow for so much more than the noise of daily existence. Once you enter the silence, you will discover it isn't empty at all.

## On the Mat: Listen to Your Mind

*Seated Meditation—Sukhasana*

Begin by finding a comfortable seat. Bring your attention to your breath. Gently shift your awareness to your thinking mind. Listening to the Mind Voice, simply observe what it's saying. Do not try to change it. Do not try to force it. Do not try to make it behave. Sometimes it takes a few moments of silence before you can hear her. No need to rush. Simply wait until you notice your mind drift. Continue your breath.

With open curiosity, simply watch what your mind does. Maybe it already drifted off and you didn't even notice. Maybe you're in a quieter space and you're still focused on your breath.

As soon as you hear your Mind Voice, quietly listen to it.

Ask yourself: *What is my mind talking about? What is it saying? Did I even notice that the voice was talking?*

Take a moment and write down what you heard in your journal. No need for detail, just jot down the main points. As you move through this practice, it's not necessary that you hear the exact words your Mind Voice is speaking, the intention is that you start to recognize the moment where you begin to drift off and your Mind Voice takes over. Anytime you find this happening, simply stop and record the topic in your journal and then come back to your practice. As you continue to drop into the present moment and catch your mind wandering, just come back to your journal and jot down the idea. The simple act of writing down the idea helps you to distance yourself from the Mind Voice and helps your mind let go. Sometimes acknowledging the voice of worry is enough. It will settle down once acknowledged.

Ask yourself again: *What is my mind talking about now? What is it saying? Did I even notice that the voice was talking?*

As soon as you hear the next topic, stop and take a moment to record it in your journal.

For the next few minutes, in your seated posture, close your eyes. Without too much effort and without trying to control, simply witness yourself as you inhale and exhale. Try not to have an agenda. Try not to be too rigid. This is simply an exercise in witnessing what happens as the mind drifts in and out. At any time, if you notice your mind has drifted, open your eyes and take a moment to note that in your journal. Try not to get too involved in the journaling process at this point. No matter what you end up writing down in your journal, this practice declutters your mind, helps you become aware of how your mind works, and deepens your sense of connection. Simply make a note. Leave it. And then return to your breath with curiosity as you wait for the next moment when your mind slips away.

There's no need to hold anything too tightly right now. Continue this cycle until your mind starts to become quiet. It may take four or five cycles of breathing and journaling before you notice a shift to stillness. Once you notice the stillness, allow the quiet to take up space. Notice if you can protect that space, even lengthen it.

## Off the Mat: Listen to Your Mind

Whether you're on the yoga mat, taking a walk on the beach, sitting in traffic, or having a coffee at your local café, you can practice tuning in to your Mind Voice at any time. Personally, I love keeping a journal nearby and tend to travel through my days with one near my side. It's an invaluable tool and I highly suggest you carry one as well.

There are two prerequisites for your journal. First, you must like the look, feel, and size of it. My journal is one of my most valuable possessions and after a while, I've become quite attached to my particular brand as well. Black hardback Moleskines are my favorite. No lined pages for me, I like the blank pages. The freedom and beauty that I associate with those crisp white papers, the hard, black binding, the elastic band—I get an incredible amount of joy from Moleskin journals. On my bookshelf, you'll see rows of these, with 2018, 2017, 2016, written in black Sharpie marker along the top edge of the pages. In my garage, you'll find boxes going back decades. Why so many journals? Because I keep everything in them.

Which brings me to the second prerequisite: keep only one journal at a time and write everything in it. Listen, I hear you—I know that some of you probably have a bunch of rules about what goes in a journal and what doesn't go in a journal. Maybe you have one journal for your inner thoughts and feelings and another crappy little notebook for where you keep a list of things to do. Maybe you have a different journal for uplifting quotes, notes from TED talks, or poems you love. Look, if you have a system that's already working, I'm not going to mess with it. But, is it working? Do you use your journals? Are they with you when you really need them? Do you know how to easily find what you've written?

I make a living at fine-tuning tools to help people navigate their lives. And I know that the people who succeed at creating change, the ones who make it to Point B, are the ones who practice often. This is why I suggest keeping *one* journal with you and why I suggest using it for everything. You'll use it because it's what you have with you. Whether I'm working on a podcast episode outline, doing book research, scribbling down a grocery list, or just emptying my mind—the act of bringing pen to page is a ritual that calms my Mind Voice, grounding me in the present moment. The work of the Four Voices doesn't need to be separate and special—but it does need to be practiced. Think of your journal as a place to practice connection off the mat.

Maybe writing down a to-do list doesn't seem like sacred or holy work. But this is where we start because this is where we are. Begin with whatever is in your head. Begin with whatever your Mind Voice is spinning around. Anytime you catch yourself trying to remember something, write it down. Anytime you catch yourself listing out a bunch of things that need to be done, write them down on the next page. Anytime you find yourself telling yourself stories from the past, or replaying scenarios from last weekend's visit to Aunt Agnes, write down the main points.

If you have a dedicated time to journal, even better.

Ask yourself: *What is my mind talking about now? What is it saying? Did I even notice that the voice was talking?*

With open curiosity, simply watch what your mind does. Still yourself and take a moment before you touch the blank page. Close your eyes and drop into conscious breathing. Try not to have an agenda. Just use this practice as a way to listen to what's already wanting to happen in your mind. Over time, you'll be able to look back over your pages and you'll start to see patterns. In your own handwriting, you'll begin to see how your Mind Voice shapes your life.

chapter three

# Allowing Mind to Guide You

How to use the mind's map
while you're awake in the driver's seat.

I have two friends. One is full of adventure—constantly pushing edges, taking risks, and going too fast. The other is timid and careful.

When we're in a group, my wild friend is the center of the action. He's gregarious and fun but often wants to break the rules, stay out too late, or party too hard. My timid friend is an alarmist and he's not shy about speaking up when he thinks we're doing something wrong. We rely on him to be the responsible one in the group. He's predictable and never going to be the one who goes rogue. Yet, if he becomes anxious and bossy, we don't listen to him. The louder he talks and the more he tries to control the situation, the more we ignore him.

When he gets quiet and serious, we all slow down and intently listen to what he has to say. His advice often keeps the group from careening off into irresponsible behavior. When he's calm, we trust him. When he is steady and clear, we know we should heed his advice.

This is almost exactly how it works with the Mind Voice. The Mind Voice holds an important part of the map and offers a critical piece of your inner guidance. But when the voice is active, triggered, and chaotic, its guidance isn't valuable. In a tumultuous mind, anxiety is high. This anxiety causes reactivity—the opposite of stability—rendering the Mind Voice's navigation meaningless. The mind becomes useful only when it is still. In the calm, there is space for truth to arise. Through that truth, you start to find your way.

## Sit Still

Many western and eastern traditions teach a practice of contemplation for spiritual growth—a conscious practice of stilling the mind. Patanjali's Yoga Sutra, compiled over two thousand years ago, are widely regarded as one of the authoritative texts on yoga. In Sanskrit, *sutra* translates to "thread." Patanjali's text contains 196 sutras or threads. Sutra 1.2 states, "The restraint of the modifications of the mind-stuff is Yoga."[4] This suggests that the "map" or the guidance isn't in the modifications and it's not in the busyness—it's in the restraint. The map won't be found by following the voice in your head, it'll be found in the discipline of stillness—in the calm that happens when the voice is quiet. You can cultivate this stillness through disciplined practice—through yoga, conscious breath, and meditation.

The Mind Voice is programmed to try to find safety and predictability, and anytime it is disturbed it reads the stream of information as a problem to be solved. To find stillness, you have to stop putting your Mind Voice in charge of solving your problems. This means you have to learn to *not* take the mind so seriously. When you take it seriously and react to it, it gets more active. Spiritual growth happens when you're a conscious witness to the Mind Voice, when you listen to your inner narrator, without getting lost in what it's saying. To be clear, the goal isn't to eliminate the voice—it's to listen without reaction, without attachment and without getting sucked into the mind's drama.

## False Drama

Whether you're on a yoga mat, at a work meeting, or simply getting ready in the morning, the pattern of constant, nagging mind chatter—when unchecked—can really ruin your day. The Mind Voice loves to be in charge of what's gone wrong and what needs to be improved. It wants to control all things, it wants to argue with reality. It gets busy telling you all the ways

4. Sri Swami Satchidananda, *The Yoga Sutra of Patanjali* (Buckingham, Virginia: Integral Yoga Publications, 1978), 3.

that the past is wrong and then will spend an enormous amount of energy justifying these opinions.

I once lost myself to this pattern for weeks because a woman wearing clunky wooden clogs neglected to remove her shoes and leave them in the hallway cubbies before yoga class—instead, she proceeded to walk across five rows of mats with her clogs on, set up her mat, and then walk back across our mats with her loud shoes. She then (finally) went to the cubbies, deposited her shoes, and returned to her mat. I stared at her the whole time, in utter disbelief. She had (to me) broken a very clear social contract. The fury that rose in me is now comical, ridiculous even. But at the time, I couldn't get over it. I hated her. And I hated her dumb shoe print at the top of my mat. I tore her apart in my head. I spent the entire class finding her faults, elevating my virtues, and then justifying why I was entitled to do so.

It was her fault that I had a shitty class. It was her fault that I couldn't concentrate. It was her fault that I was now in a bad mood. It was her fault that I couldn't let it go. I hated her clogs and her perky smile. I hated her perfectly manicured toenails and her wispy figure. And I didn't just stop there. Once I ran out of things to hate about her, I then found fault with the studio. I criticized the teacher for not stopping her before class, the check-in system for not teaching her how to properly enter class. I did not simply brush away the shoe print on my mat. I left it there as evidence, and stared at it between every pose.

She stepped on my mat only once, yet my Mind Voice recycled it over and over again.

The Clog Lady Incident happened years ago and I can still remember the righteous anger that pulsed through me. I cannot remember if any of my friends were in that class. I can't even remember who taught the class. But I do remember that shoe print on my mat. And I do remember my disdain for that woman.

The day I lost my mind over the clog-wearing-yogi was smack dab in the middle of one of the most difficult times in my life. I was in the middle of a brutal legal battle. I felt very alone in the world and was absolutely terrified. I felt like the entire world was against me and the only thing I had left was my yoga practice. I didn't realize it in the moment, but my desperation to feel some sense of safety colored almost everything I did. The clog-wearing-yogi triggered a deep panic and rage response in me (my little almonds went into hyperdrive). Of course, these feelings really had nothing to do with Clog Lady.

And this didn't just go on for a single class. The following day, my mind continued on its ranting, hoping to solve the problem of Clog Lady. I set up my yoga mat in the same place almost hoping that she'd do it again. When she came in wearing those clogs that I'd grown to loathe, I stared at her, sending hate vibes her way. Again, she traipsed across rows of mats with her damned clogs, narrowly missing mine, rolled out her mat, and then walked back to the cubbies to put away her shoes. Again, I spent the entire class spewing hate toward this woman in my mind.

Trying to mentally light people on fire with the power of your hateful thoughts is pretty much the opposite of finding stillness. It's the opposite of having a calm mind. And it's what can happen when you take your mind too seriously.

There's no amount of mental activity that's going to change someone's past behavior. Your mind isn't a judge and jury, or a time machine. No matter how many times your mind circles around something that is happening, you can't alter the course of someone else's behavior by wishing it so. And, no matter what's happened, your mind's constant narration of events will never change history, make someone behave, or control reality. You merely lose enormous amounts of time and energy in your mental drama.

I spent weeks of my life criticizing this woman, completely believing what my Mind Voice was telling me: if only she behaved differently, I could feel better. If only reality were different, I would feel better.

I didn't realize I had a choice. I didn't know that there was another way. I couldn't see then that my lack of compassion for a stranger in a yoga studio—and my anger and disdain—were evidence of my mind's power to distract me from emotional pain. I might have pulled back a little from my mind and seen that the almonds were trying to do their job to make me feel safe, but they were radically failing. I might have seen that I was grasping at pseudo-power—mentally tearing Clog Lady apart—rather than doing the difficult work of going within and dealing with my severe sense of powerlessness. If I'd had the discipline to still my mind, for even a moment, I might have stopped taking every stray thought so seriously. I may have even found a moment of inner peace. A moment where the world—in all of its brutal chaos—had permission to be as-is.

## One True Thing

If the goal is to stop taking it all so seriously, how do you do that? How exactly do you still the mind and disengage from the disturbances?

One of my favorite quotes on writing is from Hemingway's memoir, *A Moveable Feast*. In the book, he mentions what he'd say to himself if he found himself stuck, unable to get a story going. He offered, "All you have to do is write one true sentence. Write the truest sentence that you know." [5]

This advice is profound, not only for writers, but for anyone lost in the process of living. The Mind Voice is erratic, confusing, and contradictory. It's busy and wandering and constantly talking. It uses an enormous amount of energy pinging from one thing to the next. It's wobbly, imbalanced, and repetitive. If you typed up all of your thoughts in a twenty-four-hour period, you'd have a lot of random nonsense, a lot of fear and worry and judgment. Sorting through thousands of thoughts and grievances and worries, what one thought would you keep as true?

When imbalanced, a child's toy top careens across the floor, teetering and banging into things until it totters over. When left unattended, the Mind Voice is similarly erratic, rocky, and unstable. To stabilize the top, you have to find its sweet spot—its axis. Spinning on its axis, it stays upright and steady.

Truth is a sweet spot for the mind, an axis, a point of stabilization. It gives your mind a focus, creating a sense of calm, harmony, and safety. It gives the mind something to hold on to, something to trust. One true sentence has the power to calm the mind. Focusing on one true thing, you find stillness.

In the Clog Lady example, one true thing might have been the sentence: *I feel powerless.*

5. Ernest Hemingway, *A Moveable Feast* (New York: Charles Scribner's Sons, 1964), 22.

This was true for me at the time. Even now, years after the fact, I can feel my shoulders relax with this sentence. I can feel my mind slow down. Even now, in this moment, *I feel powerless* is true for me. This truth offers me solid ground to stand on. Notice that it's not a positive, feel-good, bright and shiny thing to say. It was simply the truth in that moment. To an extent, it is also true in this moment because it reminds me that I'm not in charge of the universe and that I can surrender to reality. If I could have found that sentence, I would have spared myself weeks of agitation. But even now, years later, this truth brings me a sense of peace.

Another possible truth in that moment: *A woman wearing shoes stepped on a yoga mat.*

Sometimes just taking the story to the bare-bone facts helps to alleviate the charge and helps you to see how ridiculous and manic your mind has become.

Another possible truth in that moment: *This is yoga.*

I was *in* a yoga class, right? It's like I missed the entire point of what I was doing. This sentence may have brought me back to the practice of connection, reminding me that in that moment, I had the opportunity to stay on my mat, but also to stay connected—to stay in community with the others in the room. To breathe.

One true thing, even when the truth isn't pretty, helps still the restlessness. By giving your mind a point of focus, you remember that you are the driver and that the mind is merely a passenger. You remember that you are not just your mind, you're the one listening to its voice.

## On the Mat: One True Thing

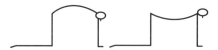

*Cat-Cow—Marjariasana /Bitilasana*

Grab a journal and pen and come to a tabletop position on all fours. Do five full rounds of Cat-Cow, inhaling as you drop your belly and lift your chin, exhaling while you round your back toward the ceiling. After completing five rounds, push back to Child's Pose. Bring awareness to the Mind

Voice. Whether it's quiet or busy, stay alert as a neutral observer and do not follow the path of thoughts. Remain in the driver's seat and watch the voice without reacting to it.

Ask yourself: *What is one true thing in this moment? What is the truest thing I know in this moment?*

When you ask yourself these questions, you might notice that your mind bounces around at first, trying to find the perfect true statement. You might notice that the mind wants to scan its archives, or that these questions agitate it. If this happens, don't worry, this is perfectly normal. Just gently bring yourself and your Mind Voice back to right here and right now. Bring yourself back to the room you're in, to the sounds around you, to the floor below you. With compassion, bring yourself back to your mat.

Drop back to Child's Pose, then ask yourself the questions again.

Ask yourself: *What is one true thing in this moment? What is the truest thing I know in this moment?*

Once you've found a true statement, record it in your journal. Maybe you found a truth about the physical space you're in: *I can feel the oak floors beneath the yoga mat.* Or a truth about the pose: *Cat-Cow feels great in my body.* Maybe you found a truth about your emotional state: *I am scared.* Maybe you found a truth about a situation: *My feelings are hurt.* Whatever truth you hear, record it in your journal and notice what happens to you as you focus on this truth.

Once you've found one true thing, come back to all fours and go through another cycle of five Cat-Cows. After five rounds, drop back to Child's Pose once again.

Ask yourself: *What is one true thing in this moment? What is the truest thing I know in this moment?*

Do not let your mind run wild here. Discipline the Mind Voice to stay on one true thing. If your mind feels unstable and wobbly, visualize the axis of a toy top and focus your mind on one true thing. Notice that one true thing might show up as a simple, basic idea.

*I am alive.*

*I am breathing.*

*This is Child's Pose.*

*I am okay.*

*I can do this.*

*I am here.*

As you continue this practice, you might begin to notice that one true thing is always available to you. As you move deeper and deeper into the truth, you might find your breathing has changed, your body's sensations have changed. You might find you've entered into a rooted sense of peace. Truth does this for the mind. In truth, you find stillness.

Continue this cycle of Cat-Cows followed by Child's Pose and journaling for three more rounds. Each time you arrive in Child's Pose, come back to one true thing, and record your truths in your journal. Once you have finished, observe and record any changes you experienced emotionally, mentally, and physically.

## Off the Mat: One True Thing

Let's say you're hosting an outdoor dinner party this evening. You've invited the neighbors and a few friends. You just finished your landscaping project and you're looking forward to utilizing your beautiful outdoor space. As the day goes on, dark clouds have started to gather on the horizon and you've become agitated. You don't want it to rain. You don't want to have to move the party indoors. Before you know it, you're nitpicking at your husband, your kids, shouting orders at them, "Clean the house, pick up your socks, go make your bed. Hurry!" You're snippy when your friend calls on the phone, saying, "I don't have time to deal with this right now." The stress level goes up and up as you scan all the things about reality you don't like.

Now, notice how I described this. I said, "*You* don't want it to rain. *You* don't want to move the party indoors." The first step in this work is to recognize that it's not *you* who's saying this in your head. It's actually only *part* of you that cares about this. Only part of you is agitated by this. Only part of you is snippy. The important thing to remember is that there's a *you* in there that's still okay and she's the one driving the car. If Mind sees the clouds and has become upset, you can work with her. You can offer her one true thing, you can calm her down. If Mind had an agenda and has noticed that it's not going her way, she might want to start arguing. She might even throw a fit. She might try to jump in the front seat and take the wheel. As long as you stay in the driver's seat, you can work with her. Through your consistent presence, you can ask her to find one true thing. And then another. And then another.

Maybe the truth sounds like: *There are clouds in the sky.*

Maybe it sounds like: *I am not in charge of the weather.*

Maybe it sounds like: *I don't need to control this.*

And as you go deeper and deeper into the truth, Mind might settle down into stillness. In this stillness, there is peace. This peace doesn't depend on the weather, and it doesn't depend on reality following Mind's rules. This peace comes from a deeper sense of self; it comes from connection and presence with life itself.

# chapter four

# When Mind Takes Over

How to wake up and chart your course
when Mind has taken the wheel.

Imagine what would happen if you verbalized everything you heard in your head. Imagine that instead of keeping your incessant mental dialogue private, you said everything out loud. People on the sidewalk would probably grab their child's hand and quickly cross the street to avoid you. At the very least, most people would politely step away from you. The line between being socially acceptable and alarmingly deranged might very well be the difference between the Mind Voice staying in your head or being broadcast loudly enough for those around you to hear.

But does the privacy of your own head make the voice any less deranged?

The answer is no. The voice is irrational. It is overly emotional, reactive, and absurd. We keep it tucked away in the privacy of our heads for good reason. When you remember this, you're able to deal with your mind pretty well. When you forget this, you can easily lose your sense of self, confusing who you are with the voice in your head.

## Beyond the Mind Voice

If you're not the voice in your head, then who are you?

There is a *you* in there—beyond the thinking voice, beyond emotion, beyond the body. This *you* has been there all along. This *you* is who you really are—your essence, your true nature. She is the watcher, the observer, the witness to all of it.

This self is not your thinking mind—she's more mysterious and marvelous than the voice your little almonds could ever dream up. This self is not your emotions—yet she has the ability to experience your emotional state. This self is not your physical body—yet she experiences life from the perspective of having a body. This self isn't your soul—but she can call on your soul for guidance.

When I talk about who you are, your true nature, your truest self, I'm talking about the part of you that has the ability to observe, inquire, relate to, and ultimately lead the Four Voices. I'm not just talking about a part of you, I'm talking about the you who integrates all parts of you together. You might call this the best you, or the you who lives most fully. Many of us only have glimpses of this self—it feels like living a very large truth—but when we allow her to lead her own Mind, Heart, Body, and Soul, she knows the way.

We sometimes find it easier to recognize this in another person we admire—this integrated sense of self. Until we integrate all the noisy parts of ourselves, we are often torn in different directions, and living halfway, or half-honest lives; we are fractured, and lost and torn. We don't have to live in the turmoil of internal chaos—we can choose the large truth of ourselves and embrace who we were always meant to be. To practice yoga is to be in conversation with that true self, to hear the true calling of who we are.

## Stillness Beyond the Voice

The word *yoga* refers to a spiritual discipline supported by a physical practice of breathing, meditation, and sequences of postures. But it also means a sense of connection, an elevated way of being part of something greater than the self. You've probably already had experiences like this, moments where you arrived so fully in yourself that the mind becomes virtually speechless—where the quieting of this voice opens you up to a profound stillness. Maybe you've experienced something like this when you witnessed a spectacular sunset—the pinks and golds and clouds and birds all doing their part to create something beyond what language can express.

Maybe for a moment, you sat there and took it in, feeling a deep connection not only to your own self but to the sunset, the birds, the ocean, the waves, to the people watching the sun go down next to you, to all the people who came before you, to some primordial sense of beauty that has been awakened in that moment.

Maybe you've experienced this sense of deep connection to the moment in an acute emergency where all the internal drama dropped away and you knew exactly what to do in that moment. In the intensity of the situation, you may have felt like time slowed, interactions became more meaningful, every second may have become precious and laden with a poignant sense of compassion.

Yoga, both on and off the mat, is meant to lead you toward living life in this way—connected to the deepest and most essential part of you. It's meant to lead you toward living life with your truest self being fully awake at the wheel. At first you might just experience this as a brief blip on the mat—maybe for just a moment you find yourself falling into a heightened sense of being. Maybe you experience a moment that feels sacred, or unexpectedly serene. Maybe you just notice an accidental astonishment, a sense of wonder and awe that can't be explained. This is what it's like to connect with your deepest sense of self—you experience the brilliance and grandeur that is life in all of its magnificence. This doesn't mean that life becomes a series of sunsets and miracles, it's more that you find yourself deeply connected to the beauty of life even in the most ordinary of moments. Instead of being caught up in the drama of your mind, you might notice the golden color of the afternoon sunlight streaming in the window. Instead of replaying a conversation that didn't go well, you might notice the warmth of the water as you wash dishes. Instead of being lost in your head, you might notice a sense of being meaningfully connected to a person standing near you in the grocery store.

When you are connected, awake and present, you know where you are, where to go, and what to do. But when you're distracted, unconscious, or sleepwalking through life, you forget who you are.

Wayfinding work is to stay present and awake. When you're awake, it's easier to remember who you are. It's easier to hear the Mind Voice and to see it as a separate entity—a voice derived from little almonds that are wanting to keep you safe. But, when life becomes uncomfortable, busy, or hectic—you might want to check out, numb out, or close your eyes and skip the hard parts. When you get upset or triggered, those almonds might scream so loud that you can no longer differentiate that voice from your own. Over time, you might become so accustomed to the chatter that you forget altogether who you are—you think that the Mind Voice is actually your own voice—you lose your *self*—and your mind takes over.

## Be Here Now

*Be here now.* You might have heard this advice offered to you during meditation, or maybe you've seen it on your mindfulness app, or heard it repeated during your community yoga class. It's the title of the ground-breaking bestseller by spiritual teacher and clinical psychologist Ram Dass, and it's one of the most popular slogans, mottos, and mantras within New Age circles. Its wide usage sometimes dilutes its message, but if you take a moment to consider these three words, you'll discover a powerful tool. This tool can immediately release you from Mind's grip and deliver you back to awareness, presence, and connection—opening a cathedral of stillness within you.

This opening of stillness might be a brief moment of liberation or a sigh of relief. It might be an abiding feeling of well-being or a flutter of levity. It might even be a poignant recognition of a sense of deep sadness or loss. Within the cathedral of stillness, you simply experience yourself as you are. When you can *be here now*—you can tap into life itself at any moment—this is the sacred connection of being alive.

This sacred connection is lost when your mind takes the wheel. When she's steering your life, you lose awareness of three important aspects: the ability to know what's real, the ability to know where you are, and the ability to know what time it is.

## Be

When you are present and connected, you find that most of your disturbances come from reacting to the Mind Voice. When Mind is in charge, the line between what's real and what's unreal becomes blurred. Mind is threatened by what it perceives to be real. Busy trying to keep you safe, Mind creates a world that can be controlled, is predictable, and is secure. It creates a world where people behave the way you'd like them to behave, where life goes your way, where you are the better/new/improved version of yourself, and where you don't have to experience the vulnerability of being human. The mind chases this fantasy world, not knowing that it's a mirage—a destination impossible to reach.

The first step back to sanity is to *be*. *Be*. This means you stop doing whatever you're doing. This means you still yourself enough to be able to perceive reality as it is actually presenting itself. Maybe this means you come back to conscious breath. *Be* breathed. *Be* grounded. *Be* available to reality. *Be* open to life as-is. Maybe this means you simply stop and notice the absurdity of your behavior. Maybe this means you take a deep breath and consciously separate yourself from the illusion playing out in your head. No matter how you do it, the goal is to arrive in a place of being—stopping all activity, ceasing to engage with the mind's delusion.

## Here

When you don't know what's real and what's unreal, your idea of location becomes problematic. You can't tell the difference between a real place or a make-believe place. When Mind is driving, you're completely cut off from your inner global positioning system—rendering any attempt toward your Point B completely worthless. You no longer have access to reality informing you of where you are on planet Earth. Your mind only sees its projected location: the destination it's chasing or the destination it's fleeing.

When you've lost your awareness of what's real, your ability to differentiate location within space becomes fuzzy and can actually be quite comical. The second step to bring you out of the mind's delusion is to come *here*. *Here*. That means you look around and notice where you are in reality. Start big: like universe big, or solar system big, or planet Earth big. Then narrow it down. Use your mind to move from make-believe into reality by zooming into your location slowly. Maybe notice if you're in the Northern or Southern Hemisphere. Then move to the continent, country, or island where your body is presently standing. Then move to town, city, or neighborhood. Then specify the location by address or park name or beach name or trail name. When you're *here*, everything is as it should be.

## Now

One of the easiest ways to recognize that Mind is steering your life, is that you don't know what time it is. The Mind exists in two time zones: the past or the future. When Mind is steering your life, it refuses to believe that it's 5:49 a.m. on a Friday morning. Rather, it's either in a make-believe alternate reality of what's going to happen next—the future. Or it's in its illusory time machine working on what already happened—the past. This symptom of the mind is chronic and widespread—if you look around, you'll see evidence of it everywhere.

One of the most recognizable ways this shows up is in waiting. By definition, waiting means that something else in the future is going to happen. If you're waiting in line, or waiting in traffic, or waiting for the video to load, or waiting for the show to start—this means that you've forgotten what time it is. Mind's idea of the future has become more important than right now. When there's no illusion of future, and only this actual moment, waiting can't happen. You're just sitting, standing, or lying down—*now*.

The other common mistake is to believe in Mind's ability to change the past. Mind does not have access to a time machine. She wants you to forget what time it is. She wants to make things safe and predictable, so she creates a fantasy past where you have ultimate history-changing powers. Anytime you're caught thinking shoulda-woulda-coulda, you might be caught in this cycle. Something happened last Sunday and you mull it over. You wish you had said something different. You wish you had behaved in a different way. This means you've forgotten what time it is. It means that Mind is at the wheel.

Connection requires a firm commitment to reality. This means you surrender the mind's time zones and inhabit only this moment. This means you become fully aware of what time it is—*now*. In the present moment—now—there might be uncomfortable emotions or sensations. But without the mind's story of a future or a past, you only experience this moment right here. You don't try to run away from what's happening right now, you simply experience it as is. In the present moment—now—there might be pleasurable emotions or sensations. Without the mind's story of a future or past, you experience them without attaching to them. You don't try to keep them or hoard them, you no longer have fear that you are going to lose anything. You simply have this moment. And then the next one. And then the next. *Now* transports you to the time zone you actually inhabit. *Now* brings you back to where real connection happens.

## On the Mat: Be Here Now

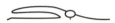

### Child's Pose—Balasana

Grab your journal and pen and come to Child's Pose for a few minutes. If your mind starts to wander, simply allow it. This practice is intended to help you notice when you shift to your Mind Voice and to help facilitate returning to connection.

After a few cycles of breath, observe your mind. Notice if you've left your sense of connection. Notice if your Mind Voice has become active.

Ask yourself: *What's real? Where am I? What time is it?*

Record your observations in your journal.

Bring your attention back to your Child's Pose. Come back to your conscious breath. Back to your practice.

Ask yourself: *What's real? Where am I? What time is it?*

Record your observations in your journal.

The practice is to *be here now*. But maybe you don't want to be here now. Maybe there are ten million things you don't like about here, or now, or being. Maybe you'd rather be doing something else, anything else other than practicing this tool, in Child's Pose.

Believe me. I get it. But I also know that giving into a tantrum like this is a shortcut to hell.

Wayfinding work isn't easy. It's not *supposed* to be easy. It's formidable to try to wrangle yourself into being in a moment that sucks. It's hard work to still yourself into somewhere you don't want to be. It's so much more convenient to go to sleep in the backseat and let someone else steer for a while.

So, sometimes you have to call on all the discipline you can muster to get yourself to do this work for even a moment.

And you're not going to want to.

Do it anyway.

And you're going to be mad at me for saying that you have to do it anyway.

Do it anyway.

Sometimes you won't have a moment of sacred stillness, or feel any shift toward your own divine nature. I wish I could tell you that the heavens will always open or that cherubs will dance around your head. I wish I could tell you anything that might convince you that doing this difficult work is worth it.

But I can't because that's not how it works.

Sometimes, you'll merely get to a point where you rail against reality a little less. Where your tantrum becomes a smidge shorter. Where reality's bite has just a little less sting. And even though it won't be rainbows and unicorns, it will be enough. *Being here now* is always enough.

This work isn't glamorous. Most of the time, it doesn't even feel that good. Sometimes, it's merely about making it through a mundane afternoon without running out of the building screaming at the top of your lungs. And that is enough.

Truly. That is enough.

## Off the Mat: Be Here Now

While cooking dinner one evening, the flood of sunlight through my kitchen windows began to blush. The days were getting shorter, fall was around the corner, and I could smell the subtle hint of wood fire smoke. I can't see the ocean from my house, but when the sunlight shifts into shades of rose and gold, I know that a spectacular sunset is in progress. I live close enough to the beach to hear the cry of seagulls as they come and go, and the hush of ocean waves are a constant soundtrack to my life. I grabbed the leather jacket and cashmere scarf that hang on pegs near the front door and hurried down to witness the last remaining minutes of the day.

On any given day, this beach is classically beautiful: white sand, pale blue water, families playing near the water with their sweet dogs. It's what you picture when you imagine a California beach.

That night, though, was breathtaking. Across the sky was a riot of color: saffron, copper, fuchsia, and magenta. Both the sky and the water seemed to be lit from deep within. Aquamarine waves of water and light folded gently toward the beach in long lines. A tangerine streak of oily sunlight spilled across the glassy sea toward the horizon. Geese in V-shape, a black silhouette against the sky's canvas, flew in formation—knowing exactly where to go. Pelicans, elegant in flight, skimmed across the tops of the waves.

In a moment like this *being here now* is effortless. The beauty of the moment has its own gravity, pulling you toward a grander cosmic connection—for which the mind has no defense. All down the water's edge, dozens of people stood in silence—all facing west, stilled by the stunning sunset.

As I stood at the water's edge, I asked myself three questions. In this moment of exquisite stillness, my answers reflected a looseness, a lightness, and probably the closest thing to true connection that day.

*What's real?* Maybe all of this and maybe none of this. The beauty. The light. The birds. The ocean. It was breathtaking. All of these things were just being themselves. The waves were doing what they do. The birds were flying where they fly. The earth was turning and the sun was setting and for a moment, I got to see those colors splashed across the sky.

*Where am I?* At the edge of the Pacific Ocean. I was standing on the cold wet sand. I was here. Only here.

*What time is it?* I didn't care. It was all-time and no-time. It was every sunset that has ever happened and it was the last sunset I might ever see. It was just simply: Now.

As you move throughout your life, you may find moments that open you to stillness, that invite you into the majesty of that particular place and time. Be aware of these moments. At those points, you might find that it's easy to *be here now.* In moments like these, you don't have to practice. Being present, being calm and connected feels natural. Make a note of how that feels: to *be here now.*

Ask yourself: *What's real? Where am I? What time is it?*

Invite whatever comes. In the moment, beauty awaits.

# Wayfinding with Your Mind Voice

To find your own way, you start by looking within through the practice of inquiry. This art of asking questions helps to clarify the message of each voice. It helps you to understand the meaning, advice, or direction that the voice offers you. Once you have a general understanding of the voice's message, you can use its wisdom for navigation.

The Mind Voice isn't a voice that's going to offer you straightforward advice. Its message will often be the voice of fear, control, powerlessness, and panic. This doesn't mean its message isn't valid. Even though it's often infused with the intention of creating a stable, predictable, and safe environment. Through inquiry, you can drop beyond the surface or reactive quality of Mind's message to find a deeper truth.

## Mind Inquiry Method

*What's the situation?*

Whether you're wanting to clarify a difficult situation, get to your version of Point B, make a decision, or find your way when you're entirely lost— start with articulating your situation. In just a sentence or two, write a short version of your dilemma, quandary, story, or situation.

*Clear the clutter.*

In Japanese cleaning consultant Marie Kondo's best-selling book, *The Life-Changing Magic of Tidying Up,* she sets forth detailed guidance to help you clear your clutter and experience the peaceful joy of living in a tidy home. Her method starts with putting your stuff in a pile, picking up each item in your hands, and then discarding what no longer sparks joy.[6] To use your mind for navigation, start with a similar approach.

First, set a timer for five minutes and dump everything from your mind onto a page. Write down everything that Mind wants to say. Don't censor and don't judge. Just allow all of the thoughts to spill onto the page. Maybe your mind offers up a list of pros and cons. Good. Write them down. Maybe your mind offers up a tirade of fear, resistance, or ridiculousness. Good. Get it all down on paper. Just let Mind speak without inhibition and record all of the thoughts. Allow it to have a voice, to have a say in the process.

Through this process of listening and recording, your mind might start to slow down. Clear out all the clutter and get it onto the page. This becomes the pile of thoughts you will now sort through.

*Throw away anything without prana.*

The Sanskrit word for life force or vitality is *prana.* In yoga philosophy, prana is not limited to animate objects but also permeates the intangible world. This pile of sentences, your mental clutter, now needs to be sorted. Most of it is trash: random nonsense that has no life force or vitality. It's unusable and uninteresting—it has no prana. Sentence by sentence, consider the thought—hold it in your mind. Toss any thoughts that feel dead, lifeless, or irrelevant. Keep thoughts and ideas that have prana—anything with a really strong emotional charge or energy associated with it.

As you mentally search through your clutter stack, prana might feel like an *ouch,* or a *hmm,* or a *that's true.* It might even seem like that particular

---

6. Marie Kondo and Cathy Hirano, *The Life-changing Magic of Tidying Up: The Japanese Art of Decluttering and Organizing* (Berkeley: Ten Speed Press, 2014), 39–42.

idea lights up, or has more punch. Put a star by anything that feels alive in this way.

### What is Mind's advice?

Now that you have been honest about what your fears are, take a look at all the thoughts that sparked interest, curiosity, or had some sense of charge to them. Here, you are looking for bright lights in the darkness, glimmers of what you really, really want underneath all the worry. What is it that Mind wants you to do? Write down Mind's advice in a short clear sentence.

### Specify your Point B for this particular situation.

Think about the big picture and articulate your larger intention, focus, commitment, and priority. Please know that your mind's advice typically won't be the most enlightened point of view, but it is a crucial piece of the puzzle, and it deserves to voice its opinion.

### Is Mind's advice taking you to where you want to go?

Considering your Point B, decide if Mind's advice will get you where you really want to go. Remember that the mind defaults toward safety, predictability, and stability. Often this tilt is at odds with your bigger desire. The things our mind warns us about may be real or unreal. But once we determine what's real, we can take conscious action.

### Thank Mind and move her to the backseat.

Remember that you are the driver of your life. Mind has valuable input, but she is not the driver. Consider her advice and then determine your course of action or your next step from the larger point of view—that of your whole self.

Here's your new script: "Thank you, Mind, for trying to protect me from _____. Sometimes this is impossible to completely avoid but I appreciate your input. My larger intention, focus, commitment, and priority is _____. Therefore, I will _____."

# Quick Review of the Mind Inquiry Method

1. What's the situation?

2. Clear the clutter. Write it all down.

3. Throw away anything without prana.

4. What is Mind's advice?

5. Specify your Point B for this particular situation. There is power in naming, and in writing down new beliefs or directions. The truth on the page is so much more real than a passing hope you don't even bother to write down.

6. Is Mind's advice taking you where you want to go? Is the pattern in your thinking sending you repeatedly into a brick wall, or are your thoughts helping you to imagine a better future?

7. Thank Mind and move her to the backseat. Whether your mind is a worrywart today or a benevolent creator, say thank you.

*Example: Spinning in Overwhelm*

1. **What's the situation?** I'm feeling deeply overwhelmed and consumed with self-doubt as I sit down to finish a project. I don't know how to keep going.

2. **Clear the clutter.** List of thoughts: *This is too hard. I'm never going to get this done. I'm going to lose my friends and family. I'm not going to get far. I'm going to go broke. I'm going to have to completely trash everything I've written anyway. It won't be good enough. I'm going to have to start over. All of this work is going to be for nothing. I don't have any good ideas. I'm running out of time.*

3. **Throw away anything without prana.** After mentally picking each thought up to get a feel for it, the thought with the most life in it was *This is too hard.*

4. **What is Mind's advice?** Stop. Give up. You're not good enough.

5. **Specify your Point B for this particular situation**. My Point B is to completely finish the project, to keep going, and to deliver the product by deadline.

6. **Is Mind's advice taking you to where you want to go?** No. My greater intention is to complete the project. That's my Point B. If I take Mind's advice, I will not get to Point B.

7. **Thank Mind and move her to the backseat.** "Thank you, Mind, for trying to protect me from *possible future pain*. Sometimes this is impossible to completely avoid but I appreciate your input. My larger intention, focus, commitment, and priority is *to finish this project*. Therefore, I will *disregard your advice*."

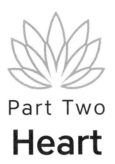

Part Two
# Heart

The heart's voice is subtle and often wordless. The heart translates our experiences into emotions, and if we are listening, we *feel* rather than hear our path forward. In the succeeding chapters, I'll show you how the heart works. I'll show you what happens when you are connected and use the Heart Voice for navigation, how each feeling offers you feedback and guidance. I'll also show you what happens when you can't handle your heart and try to silence it and what happens when you jump in the backseat and let Heart drive your life.

chapter five

# The Heart Voice

An introduction to the voice of the heart.
How it works, how to recognize it,
and how it influences your journey.

For most of my life, I was severely out of touch with my feelings. On the outside, I was stoic and able to handle almost anything life threw at me. On the inside, I spent almost all of my waking energy suppressing constant emotional pain. Of course, I didn't know this. I had myself duped just as much as everyone around me. My childhood was riddled with violence and abuse, and I learned early on not to let anyone around me know what I was feeling. Showing fear, anger, or any other emotion was like throwing gasoline on the fire of rage. During episodes of abuse, I'd go far, far away in my head. I'd be as silent and still as possible.

This ability to compartmentalize kept me safe and probably saved my life as a child. But as I matured into adulthood, I didn't know how to not compartmentalize. It wasn't until I gave birth to my daughter—and for the first time in my life, I felt unconditional love—that the drawers and drawers of little boxes in my head started to dump out all their feelings, flooding my nights with panic and an overwhelming sense of doom. I lost the ability to sleep as the tidal wave of all of the painful emotions that I'd buried long ago threatened to take me under. My sweet little girl had broken my heart wide open and there was no turning back. I could no longer keep everything in the boxes. So I began the decade-long journey to reclaim my heart, to learn how to feel and how to stop numbing, avoiding, and running from my emotions.

At first, my only access to the Heart Voice was that I knew if I felt really bad or if I felt less bad. I was either drowning or just exhausted and treading water. I had no way to distinguish variations of emotions, nor the ability to categorize them or name them. Once I could finally open my heart, I could finally start to use my feelings for navigation. If you have a history of abuse, trauma, addiction, or distraction—wayfinding with your Heart Voice might be as difficult for you as it was for me. Be patient with yourself, this isn't a race.

## What Is the Heart Voice and How Does It Work?

When I speak about the heart, I'm not referring to the tangible muscular organ that pumps blood through your body; I'm talking about the intangible gateway to the elusive inner world of emotions. This intangible heart is the portal to emotion, the epicenter of where emotions are felt, but it's also the birthplace or the spring from which they flow.

Even though the intangible heart might sound mysterious or even metaphysical, when you look at evolutionary theory there's a good deal of research that helps to explain the function, history, and intelligence of emotions. I am not an evolutionary biologist but I find it valuable to understand a little about anthropology and evolution when it comes to matters of the heart.

The Heart Voice communicates through emotions. Emotions are different than physical sensations. If you hold your hand near fire, you'll feel heat and pain. The heat and pain are not emotions, these are physical sensations. Depending on how long you hold your hand there, you'll feel varying degrees of heat and pain. This pain is a warning signal that's meant to keep you alive. If you felt no pain, you'd run the risk of mortally wounding yourself without even realizing it. This natural physical sensation of pain deters you from holding your hand to the heat for too long and the memory of that pain helps to ensure that you remember not to try to touch fire again in the future.

Similarly, if you felt no physical pleasure, you might not feed yourself, hydrate, or bear offspring. Pleasure and pain are physical sensations that keep you alive, safe, and procreating.

Emotions evolved for similar reasons. Emotional pain was meant to be felt in order to deter you from behavior that harmed you. It helped you cope with threat, avoid danger, and defend yourself. And, emotional pleasure was meant to be felt so that you'd replicate behavior that felt good—keeping you alive and ensuring your DNA would have the opportunity to reproduce. These emotions motivated you to procure food and water, seek reproductive opportunities, and find community, shelter, and safety.

## What Are Emotions and How Do They Work?

When I talk about emotion, I am referring to a reaction—conscious or unconscious—a phenomenon or physiological response that plays out in the theater of your body, a response that colors the way we experience life itself. Each emotion evolved with a distinct and clear function. Whether it was sadness, fear, anger, happiness, or guilt—each individual feeling has encoded within it a specific directive, a prescribed action. These messages are the language of the Heart Voice. Through the individual emotions, the Heart Voice offers directions to either stop doing something or to start doing something. Your feelings have a function, a job to do, a clear message behind them—just like the pain of holding your hand to the fire has a job to signal you to take your hand away from the fire.

Emotions worked beautifully in hunter-gatherer societies and in pre-industrial life. Fear kept you safe and helped you either flee or freeze. Anger helped keep warring societies from invading and hurting your young. Shame kept you from doing anything too weird that would lead to ostracism from the pack—an undoubtable death sentence. These feelings had functions, they were felt in real time, they offered clear direction, and they had very short life spans. They evolved to be short lived and last only about ten to fifteen seconds because any longer than that would have gotten in the way of survival.[7]

But now fear keeps you up for hours at night worrying about a stupid comment on Instagram—you can't freeze in the online world and there's nowhere to flee so fear just spins out of control with no real way to get you to safety. Anger is no longer honored as critical protection—now we're taught to manage it, stuff it, or repress it—rendering its power impotent. Shame no longer protects us because there's no way to ever feel like you belong when there's no actual community to belong to.

You're now bathing for hours, days, years, in painful emotions that were supposed to give you a quick fifteen seconds of feedback. What used to be a signal to motivate you to take action has now deteriorated into an amorphous blob of suffering. And now you suffer without knowing what to do because these signals are muddy and convoluted, and not easily understood. This confusion compounds upon itself, creating a crushing amount of emotional pain in your everyday life.

Imagine that, if instead of taking your hand away from the hot stove, you were taught to just hold it there and ignore what you felt. Imagine if over time you got better and better at not feeling the pain from the fire, not listening to your body's wisdom. Imagine if over time, you simply repressed, numbed, stuffed, denied, ignored, and neglected the pain.

Imagine how many beers you'd have to drink, how many cookies you'd have to eat, or how many episodes of *The Office* you'd have to binge-watch to numb the torture of having your hand continually held to the fire.

Over eons, the human race evolved to feel feelings, to listen to the feedback they offered, and to quickly *do* something with the information. Emotions are biologically rooted, part of our evolutionary history and universal across cultures. But over the last couple of hundred years, modern society has done everything it can to ignore the Heart Voice and numb its feedback—rendering humans artificially incapacitated. We live a life of holding ourselves to the emotional fire because we are not listening to the Heart

7. June Gruber, "Human Emotion 4.1: Evolution and Emotion, Yale University," filmed May 2013. YouTube video 21:14, posted May 2013, https://www.youtube.com/watch?v=fH-azxAhU-I.

Voice, and we've forgotten how to speak its language. We live life deaf to a voice that evolved to protect us and to help us to thrive and connect—a voice that evolved to give us clear direction. And this deafness has created a landslide of problems.

## The Language of the Heart Voice

The Heart Voice speaks in the language of emotions. These emotions or feelings evolved to help you meet challenges of particular situations. They are a response to events and are meant to facilitate your survival, or the survival of your group and species. They help motivate you to care for your children, navigate social hierarchies, create long-term bonds with partners and communities, and instill in you compassion for others. Emotions are an essential bridge of connection.

The Heart Voice speaks directly through emotions and indirectly through mood states. Mood states are feelings that last well beyond fifteen seconds. These can be a compilation of emotions that have been kept artificially alive through rumination, numbing, avoidance, or distraction.

In her TED talk, *The History of Human Emotions*, Tiffany Watt Smith said, "Emotions are not simple reflexes, but immensely complex, elastic systems that respond both to the biologies that we've inherited and to the cultures that we live in now. They are cognitive phenomena. They're shaped not just by our bodies, but by our thoughts, our concepts, our language."[8] Among theorists, there's no agreed-upon order of operations between cognition, emotion, and physiology—thought, feeling, and physical manifestations—Mind Voice, Heart Voice, and Body Voice. Sometimes the Mind Voice speaks and the Heart Voice responds. For instance, if your mind starts running scary scenarios, the heart responds with the emotion of fear. Sometimes, the emotion of fear arises in the heart first and then the Mind Voice gives a mental explanation. Sometimes the Body Voice speaks first with shivers and panic, and then heart registers fear and the mind responds with a story like, "I can't go up on stage, I'll die."

8. Tiffany Watt Smith, "The History of Human Emotions," filmed November 2017 at TED@ Merck KGaA, Darmstadt, Germany, video 14:21, https://www.ted.com/talks/tiffany_watt_ smith_the_history_of_human_emotions.

The order of operations isn't critical for the purposes of this work. What's important is that you "hear" a clear signal of fear so that you can respond to the feedback. As we move further through the voices, you'll see how intertwined they are and how often each voice is influenced by the others. This is why it's best that all Four Voices are accounted for; together, they form a trustworthy inner guidance system.

## On the Mat: Listen to Your Heart

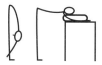

### Forward Fold and Supported Forward Fold—Uttanasana

Forward folds are, by design, introspective. By folding in on yourself, over your legs, you can practice tuning out the world and homing in on your interior sense of the intangible world of the heart. Forward folds can be calming, but only if you are supported in a way that helps you relax into the pose. Otherwise, they can bring up a slew of sensations and emotions. For this reason, you'll practice a forward fold both supported and unsupported. You will need a clock or timer and your journal and pen nearby.

To access the Heart Voice, tune in to your interior landscape to determine what you feel and then give name to the emotions you experience at any given time. Much like listening to a symphony, you can take in the overall beauty of the song or you can focus on specific instruments within the orchestra. At first, you may not hear the reedy whine of the oboe, the round warmth of the French horn, the thunder of the timpani, or the second chair violas running counterpoint to the melody as you hum along. But if you zero in on an individual musical quality, you may recognize the sound and then name the instrument playing that particular line within the song. Listening to your Heart Voice requires the same level of concentration and ability to hear smaller parts within the whole.

Before beginning the yoga practice, set your timer for two minutes.

Ask yourself: *What emotion am I feeling right now? From zero being the lowest to ten being the highest, how would I rate the intensity of this emotion?*

Make a list of as many emotions as you can find along with their corresponding intensities. Without interpretation, attachment, or story, simply record your insights in your journal. If you feel discomfort, return to the breath and continue.

When you begin to tune in to your heart, please go gently. Depending on your history, this might be frustrating or difficult for you. You might start off only being able to determine two emotions: really bad or less bad. You might tune in to your heart and quickly become overwhelmed with pain. This is normal. It's almost like your heart goes, "Thank GOD; I've been waiting to have a conversation with you." That's why I'm asking you to do this with a timer—you can do almost anything for two minutes. Consider this exercise like you would any difficult yoga pose—breathe through it, stay with it.

So now let's try it on your mat. Come to a standing forward fold.

Close your eyes and move your focus into the interior of your physical body. Notice the pace of your breath, your heart rate. As you spend more time in this pose, bring your attention to the quality of your heart.

Ask yourself: *What emotion am I feeling right now? From zero being the lowest to ten being the highest, how would I rate the intensity of this emotion?*

Notice if there are multiple emotions coming up. Which emotion feels the strongest? Try not to let Mind interpret the emotion, or find its origin, just notice the emotion and how intense it feels. You are simply being a witness to the workings of your heart.

Spend at least two minutes in this meditative forward fold before coming out of the pose to journal your insights.

Now set yourself up for a supported forward fold. Depending on your flexibility level, find a chair, a couch, a bed, or even a table you can fold onto. Find something taller than the floor that can hold and secure your upper body so you can fully relax into a forward fold. Use as many pillows or blankets as you need. The more time and care you put into setting yourself up for comfort, the more information you'll get from this. This isn't about getting a deep stretch, this is more about holding a pose of introspection while feeling completely comfortable, bolstered, and safe.

The goal of this practice isn't to try to cultivate positive feelings. The goal is to simply witness what you're really feeling. It's not to change it or to try to steer your emotions toward a better-feeling outcome. Rather, it's to listen to Heart's honest feedback. There is no bad news when it comes to the heart. Painful feelings give you just as much insight as positive feelings do. Emotions are intended to move through us, give us information, and then let go of us. When painful emotions surface, don't fight them; if you allow them to move through you, I promise they won't take up permanent residence. In the next chapter, I'll teach you what to do with those painful feelings and what specific piece of navigational advice each holds.

## Off the Mat: Listen to Your Heart

Listening to your heart works best when it's practiced both on and off the mat. To take this practice off the mat, many of my clients have found it beneficial to set an alarm that reminds them to check in. You can easily do this as a recurring alarm on your calendar, or you can set this up through an app on your phone. At several points throughout your day—I recommend three times a day—check in with yourself and try to name the emotion or emotions you feel. I recommend keeping a journal of these check-ins so you can see the trends over time. As you hone your listening skills, you'll find it becomes easier to name what you're feeling.

Similar to the on the mat practice, set your timer for two minutes.

Ask yourself: *What emotion am I feeling right now? From zero being the lowest to ten being the highest, how would I rate the intensity of this emotion?*

Record your insights in your journal.

# chapter six

# Allowing Heart to Guide You

How to use the heart's map
while you're awake in the driver's seat.

In kindergarten, I learned that the primary colors were red, yellow, and blue. I also learned that I could mix these colors together and make any other color imaginable. Emotions are kind of like that. There's a basic group of them and then—depending on how they're mixed together—you will experience countless variations and intensities of emotions throughout a single day or even a single hour. There are a few common emotions that almost every human feels (or tries not to feel) some of the time. These emotions evolved to offer specific guidance—a map that many of us, unfortunately, lost long ago when we forgot how to tap into how we really *feel*. So even though there is a full spectrum of other feelings—beautiful, terrible, exquisite, and sublime as they are—I'm going to teach what I've found to be the core wayfinding emotions so that when you're in the driver's seat of your life, you can rely on the guidance that your Heart Voice provides.

Remember when you read about pain being a signal to move your hand away from the fire? And how if you didn't feel pain, you might not move your hand, in which case you could burn your arm right off? And how emotions evolved from the same concept—to get you to *do* something for your own good? In the fire-hand-pain scenario—pain is actually doing a job: causing you to immediately remove your hand from the fire. I'd like to invite you to see emotion through this same lens: as honest, immediate feedback about what feels good and what feels bad.

## Fear

Fear is so common it's almost impossible to think about what a life might be like without it. That beige, low-grade stress in the background of your day? Fear. That anxiety that keeps your head spinning at night? Fear. That worry about missing out, not keeping up, falling behind, or that you're never going to find your true life's purpose? Fear. And fear. In all its intensities—from worry to terror—fear plays an important role in your life. Remember those little almonds in your head? Almost everything that they talk about has something to do with fear.

Fear evolved to keep you safe in situations where you're being threatened. It was meant to keep you safe from things like lions and tigers and bears and falling off of cliffs and wildfires and other acts of nature. But here's the thing about fear in our day and age: whether the predator is real or imaginary, you experience fear in the same way.

If a scary beast chases you, fear kicks in—an urgent rush that says: DANGER! Your heart pumps faster and more blood gets sent to your arms and legs (think fight-or-FLIGHT), you breathe faster and get more oxygen flowing through your body. This helps you run away, and if you can't run away, you might just duck under a bush nearby, hold your breath, and wait as quietly as possible for the beast to pass.

Unfortunately, in today's world, the types of things that freak you out were never originally encoded into this fear system. There's no way to run or hide from mortgages and taxes and the pressures of modern-day life. These things aren't chasing you—but it sure feels like they are. Modern life and all of its stress is pervasively filled with things that freak you out. So that leaves you with the same rush that says: DANGER! Your heart pumps and your body gets ready to run—but there's no real path and there's no real beast and there's not even a bush to duck under until it passes.

And it's okay, this is just fear doing its job. Once you identify fear, you can start to diffuse it—you can respond to the fear rather than emotionally holding yourself to the fire.

Fear is Heart Voice relaying the message: This is unsafe. This is danger-ous. Don't attack, RUN! HIDE!

Now, if you are being chased by a scary beast, please run. If you're not—and you know that this fear signal is probably coming from a modern-era-issue—there are a few things you can do. Fear prepares flight. It wants you to escape the predator, it wants you to get to safety. This means you're going to have to get clear about the true threat.

### What You Might Be Tempted to Do

When you're afraid, you often want to give up and give in. When you have too much of that beige anxiety fuzzy-headed static running through you all the time, you might want to just avoid the whole damned thing. You might want to just crack open a beer to make the voices stop. Giving up and giving in is the opposite of what fear is designed for. It's basically laying yourself at the foot of danger, silencing hundreds of thousands of years of evolution.

### What Not to Do

When you're really afraid, you might feel that drive to *do* something but not exactly know what to do, so you might freak out and run around in circles. You might put your head in the sand and try to ignore what's happening. You might get super hyper-vigilant and start trying to control everyone and everything around you. None of these behaviors use the wisdom garnered from fear. None of these behaviors will take you where you really want to go. You might get a quick hit of relief from the fear because you're doing something, but eventually your Heart Voice will give you more fear because the predator is still out there and you've done nothing to remove yourself from the danger.

### What You Should Do

Fear wants you to sharpen all five of your senses. This means bringing your full attention to what you see, smell, hear, taste, and the physical sensa-tions you feel. It wants your full system to be alert. (Notice that this is the exact opposite of reaching for the beer or putting your head in the sand.

Numbing and denial are polar opposite reactions and end up creating a never-ending spiral of fear.) Pay careful attention to what might be threatening your surroundings—both inner and outer. (Fear feels just as threatened by internal—emotional, spiritual, and mental threats—as it does physical.) Patrol the perimeter—keep careful watch over your (physical, emotional, and spiritual) boundaries. Clarify the specific threat and determine first if the threat is real or imaginary. (Is the fear Mind Voice driven? Is it true?) If it's imaginary, default to Mind Voice tools. If the threat is real, determine what, if any, action will ensure your safety. Do whatever you can to move yourself (or your loved ones) away from the threat.

## Guilt and Shame

I can be really creative when it comes to guilt and shame. I can feel guilty for just about anything. This guilt-super-power has followed me throughout my life and has infected almost every corner of my experience. Not eating healthy? Guilt. Not exercising enough? Guilt. Too much TV? Guilt. Not doing enough for my friends, love ones, daughter, pets, plants? Guilt, guilt and more guilt.

Over time, guilt puts you into a smaller and smaller box with more and more rigid rules. There came a point in my life when I realized that I couldn't do one single thing without guilt. I couldn't eat a single thing without guilt. I couldn't work without guilt. I couldn't parent without guilt. I couldn't rest without guilt. Every single thing that I did felt wrong, bad, not good enough.

I'm also no stranger to shame. Not smart enough. Not pretty enough. Not skinny enough. Not rich enough. Not nice enough. Shame, shame, shame, and shame. You know that hot-burning horrible sense that you're not enough, you'll never be enough and that something inside of you is intensely flawed, wrong, bad? Yep, that little darling is the feeling called shame.

Much has been said about the difference between shame and guilt. For the purposes of this work, I'm going to group shame and guilt together because their function is similar: basically to keep you from getting way off course in human relationships. Guilt is the emotion that comes up when your actions have negative effects on the well-being of others (aka: do something wrong, hurt other people, do something immoral or unethical). It's about your behavior, about a wrong action. It shows up when you did something you don't feel good about. Guilt is actually a very useful feeling for protecting the integrity of your relationships; it can direct you to changing your behavior toward others so you can strengthen and deepen your connections to others.

Where guilt comes up as a reaction to *doing something wrong or bad,* shame is about *being* or having innate qualities that are wrong or bad. Shame comes up when you feel you *are* something bad, wrong, not enough. But these two feelings feed off of each other because you can start to tell yourself that you did something bad because you are a bad person, who does wrong things because you are wrong—you get the picture?

Shame and guilt are signals to make you move away from something harmful, threatening, or dangerous. They are akin to the pain-causing flame, and are meant to give you a clear and distinct signal to keep you away from ostracism.

In pre-modern eras, shame, guilt, rejection, regret, remorse, self-consciousness, embarrassment, humiliation—all the variations found within these emotions—were early warning signs to help you stop behaving in a way that would lead to ostracism, exclusion, banishment, or exile.

In this modern age—especially in self-help-y circles—you're told to stand out from the pack. Enter the arena. Be unique. Let your freak flag fly. Nothing is wrong with this advice, I actually find it to be incredibly valuable—but it comes with a price. Outliers have to tolerate an overwhelming force that's constantly trying to get us to move right back into the middle of the pack. It's the force that's trying to keep us from losing connection with those whom we love and rely upon. This force is the shame-y-guilty pressure that we feel within, the not-good-enoughness that can stonewall our best efforts.

There's also this fun fact—once upon a time we only had to manage being not-too-weird for a small number of people. Our particular group, society, town, herd, tribe, or band of brothers was tangible. We could count these people on our fingers and toes—we knew them all by name, and we understood our role within that group. Nowadays, the social "norm" includes everybody and I do mean everybody. Or at least everybody in your neighborhood, on Facebook, on Instagram, in the movies, on TV (on all 27,813 channels), in magazines, in the newspaper, on YouTube, in the media, with a blog. I could go on. Our social group is now too large to count, and always shifting. And that's a problem because it's really hard to know the rules of the social group when the group numbers infinity.

How can we possibly try to be smack dab in the middle of a group that includes all of humanity? How can we possibly try to be the norm of beauty, talent, aging, achievement, or fitness when people such as Heidi Klum, Beyoncé, Bill Gates, or LeBron James are in our mix? How can we possibly know where the middle of ethics, morality, or goodness lies when society no longer has a central tradition? And worse than that, these superstars are not being presented as if they are indeed the outliers—marketing now pushes the idea that these outliers are the new norm, completely attainable if you just try harder, the new goal, the new middle.

And when Beyoncé, Heidi, and LeBron become the new middle—the rest of us become the strange freaky people on the edge of ostracism. No wonder you can't go bra shopping, or introduce yourself to a stranger in your yoga class, or get yourself out of the house on a Friday night without having to work through ten tons of shame.

This lack of being able to achieve the middle-ness, safeness, and belongingness makes your inner moral compass spin wildly out of control. Shame and guilt were never meant to be felt at the levels we tolerate now. They were meant to be the pain that made you pull away from the metaphorical flame. They were meant to be a signal to move toward connection, intimacy, and your group.

This is exactly the opposite of what we do now.

The very last thing I want to do if I'm feeling steeped in shame is to reach out and get all vulnerable with someone. No, thank you. I'd rather stay in darkness all alone. But this is how the shame spiral gains momentum. Instead of moving toward intimacy, we move away.

When you feel shame or guilt, the Heart Voice is saying: There's a threat of disconnection—make it right and repair the relationship. Move toward intimacy and vulnerability. Move away from the scary beast called ostracism.

### What You Might Be Tempted to Do

You might try to hide yourself away to secretly improve yourself for re-entry. You might want to just hole up somewhere until you're prettier, smarter, thinner, richer, younger—that elusive Better You that can handle all the hard things with ease. You might start giving yourself ridiculous rules about how to achieve that Better You. There's no version of you that won't have to deal with shame/guilt. It's a natural part of being human.

### What Not to Do

When you're feeling guilty or shame-y you might be tempted to go dark, to ghost out, to disappear. You'll probably want to withdraw from people you love, hide yourself, isolate and keep your shame secret. Going dark, hiding, ignoring, and isolating won't fix this and it definitely won't help you move toward the goal: connection.

You'll also probably want to think about yourself a lot. Shame and guilt are both self-conscious feelings, meaning they are about being *ultra-conscious* of *self*. This makes you focus on *you* rather than on other people. This only fuels the fire of shame. The more you think about yourself, the more you focus on what created the sense of shame or guilt. Try as much as possible to focus on someone or something you love. Break through the self-centeredness of these feelings and work toward other-ness, which automatically starts to feel more like belonging (which is the goal here).

### What You Should Do

Guilt and shame both want you to do the same thing—move toward connection, intimacy, and vulnerability. This might mean saying you're sorry, making amends, repairing damage, and owning your part. It also might mean getting really real with someone (again—you won't want to do this but do it anyway) and sharing your shame. It means moving toward someone and taking the risk to allow yourself to be seen, understood, and witnessed. This is best done with someone you love and trust.

## Anger

Stand in line at the post office, the grocery store checkout line, or the slowest moving line anywhere—the DMV—and you might get to the point where you're rolling your eyes, sighing, tapping your toes, leaning on one hip and then the other, checking the clock, sighing again—basic signs of impatience. You know that growing feeling of frustration you get when someone or something is in your way? That's anger. At home, when your spouse forgets to pick up toilet paper and you really don't want to have to go out again tonight and *ugh why do you have to do everything around here?* That's anger too. Coming out of Target, when you just don't have time to add anything else to your plate and up walks some well-meaning-dolphin-loving-clipboard-holding-survey-taker and you hold up your hand as you walk by and just try to get out of the parking lot without having to get involved in saving any part of the planet? You guessed it—anger.

Anger may be an uncomfortable feeling but it is an important and necessary emotion. The fire/flame/pain here is that something or someone is hindering your progress, keeping you from something you want, or encroaching on your territory. It is physiologically similar to fear (think FIGHT-or-flight) in that your blood flow increases to your arms and legs (for fighting) and oxygen volume increases. Your body gets ready to rumble.

Unlike shame, where you've been socialized into feeling more of it—anger is one of those dirty-little-feelings that society has tried to beat completely out of you. Since you were little, you were told to be nice, play fair, smile, make people like you, *blah blah blah*. Maybe you were told that anger is wrong, a sin, bad. Maybe you were told that angry women are bitches and angry men are assholes and you don't want to be seen like that so you've buried your anger way down deep and spent a lifetime working on your veneer of nice-ness.

Maybe you experienced the wrong end of someone with a rage issue and you've vowed to never be angry like that. If so, I'm very sorry for your experience, but that wasn't healthy anger. Healthy anger is not tyranny, intimidation, domination, or threats. It's not malevolence, cruelty, or brutality. Anger isn't about controlling another person, about hurting another person, or about wanting anyone (or anything) to suffer. Anger is about protection. Where fear is about running and hiding from threat, anger is about protecting yourself from threat.

Anger comes in many flavors—from irritation, impatience, and annoyance to wrath, exasperation, fury, and resentment. When flowing naturally, anger rises up in proportionate intensity to the threat. Small infractions are met with mild annoyance.

Anger evolved to protect us and to keep us (and our loved ones) safe. It evolved to help us protect ourselves and our community. It's a response to any situation where your goal is being thwarted or stymied. Whether someone (or something) has encroached on your boundary, or something has become increasingly unfair—anger ensures that you fight, hold your ground, and protect what's yours.

Anger wants you to do something, it wants you to take action, it wants you to speak words, move your body. Protect what's yours.

In animals, you've seen this countless times. A puppy tries to play with his mom and jumps at her, runs circles around her, nips at her feet, and basically gets all up in her space. Dog Mom bares her teeth and snarls. It's not a big deal—she's annoyed and she's signaling the puppy to back off. If the puppy doesn't listen, Dog Mom's response gets more aggressive—maybe a snarl and a bark. Still, no big deal. Puppy goes about her business and Dog Mom gets some alone time. This is what healthy, free-flowing anger looks like. It's simply a "Back it up, buddy" response to someone who's too close.

If a scary beast comes at you, and you realize that this beast isn't so big (you can take 'em)—anger kicks in—a quick rush that says: PROTECT! Your heart pumps faster and more blood gets sent to your arms and legs, you breathe faster and get more oxygen flowing through your body. This helps you call upon your strength—whether that means you yell, scream, hit the thing with a stick, or simply give it a don't-mess-with-me death stare.

Unfortunately, you've been taught this isn't *nice*. You're taught that having boundaries isn't *nice*, protecting what's yours isn't *nice*. You're taught to say *yes* to everything. You're taught to suck it up and smile. And all that healthy anger gets swallowed and silenced and pushed down farther and farther.

You know what else is nice? Staying alive. Protecting your loved ones. Fighting for what's fair. So, to allow anger to do its job, you might have to redefine *nice* for yourself. And this might bring up a bunch of fear—that's okay, you can work with fear—and then get back to anger.

Anger is Heart Voice relaying the message: Confront this problem. Someone or something is in the way of what I want. Someone is doing something wrong. I need to protect what's mine.

Now, if a beast threatens you, please protect yourself. But this doesn't mean you go postal every time you're in a grocery store line. Healthy anger isn't about taking what's *not* yours. It's not about acting unfairly. It's not about becoming a bully or a tyrant. It's not about lobbing empty threats at people, or posting angry comments on social media. That's not healthy anger. Anger is simply a "Back it up, buddy" response. It's a simple, "No, thank you," or "That doesn't work for me."

### What You Might Be Tempted to Do

You might want to get all spiritual and act like nothing's wrong. You might get caught up in trying to stay a likable, boundary-less, people-pleasing doormat. You might want to send up imaginary smoke signals hoping that the person can just simply read your mind so you don't have to say *the words* or take *the action* to protect your boundaries. You might want to use food, or alcohol, or TV, or any other distraction to keep a barrier between you and the intruder. It's okay to want to do these things—but to protect, you must act or else that irritation inside of you will eventually fester to full-blown fury.

### What Not to Do

You also might want to go the passive-aggressive route—a strategy where you don't mean what you say and you don't say what you mean. It's an indirect resistance and an avoidance of direct confrontation (the exact opposite of what anger evolved to do). It might give you some sense of relief (because people stay away), but it doesn't protect you or your loved ones.

Another passive-aggressive technique is to quietly remove yourself from the problem—spending greater and greater amounts of time reading, watching TV, gardening, or climbing mountains—anything to keep you from having to set boundaries or to protect what's being threatened. You might also use sarcasm and humor to diffuse your power rather than direct communication to protect what's rightfully yours. This isn't how anger was designed to function.

### What You Should Do

Protect what's yours. Sometimes this means risking the relationship you're trying to protect. Set healthy boundaries—meaning you protect your emotional, physical, spiritual, and financial well-being. This means getting really good at saying, "No," or "That doesn't work for me," or "Back it up, buddy." It means you stop doing things you don't want to do. It means you stop saying yes to things that threaten your well-being. It means you fight when necessary, speak your mind, and share your opinion.

## Sadness

From feeling slightly bummed or having a bit of the blues to having hurt feelings or intense feelings of sorrow, despair, heartbreak, or grief—sadness comes in many forms and a variety of intensities. When you're home alone for the eighty-fifth Friday night, eating pizza in your pajamas while the rest of the world seems to be out having a great time, making friends, falling in love, getting married, and having babies without you? That lonely, achy, outcast-y feeling? Sadness. When you really thought someone liked you—like, liked-you liked-you—and you find out that they don't, at least not in *that* way? That heartbreak-y chest-pain-y despair-y hopeless feeling? Sadness. When your mom died decades ago and you're in the vitamin aisle minding your own business until some woman passes you with your mom's signature perfume wafting behind her and for just one tiny moment it's like you just lost your mom all over again? That tidal-wave of grief-y bereft-ness that thwacks you across your gut and buckles your knees? Sadness.

Sadness is the feeling that comes up when you lose something of value. The pain is caused by clinging to something that is already gone. Sadness evolved to help you cope with letting go. Loss is supposed to be painful. Otherwise, we wouldn't try so hard to keep our loved ones safe, our social bonds healthy, and our support systems intact. Loss is tragic, it means you have invested in something you no longer have. Sadness also means you need comfort, care-taking, and help.

Sadness slows you down, it diminishes your metabolism. Even though you might experience an increased heart rate, or quicker breathing (aka: sobbing), this isn't fight-or-flight. Your body becomes lethargic, softer, and slower. Crying releases hormones and other toxins that build up during stress and also stimulates the production of natural pain-killing, feel-good hormones known as endorphins.

Sadness asks you to step away from your normal way of being. It wants you to take a pause, a time-out. It wants you to withdraw so you can process the loss so you can come back to your life rejuvenated, renewed, and restored.

You had it right when you were a baby. You cried and screamed and elicited all sorts of sympathy when you needed comfort. You knew you needed to be held. You knew you needed help. But then you had to grow up and you were most likely taught not to cry in your crib or wait for people to attend to your needs. You were probably taught to stop complaining, to hide your sadness, to stop feeling all those messy feelings, and to stop being so damned sensitive. To try to survive without your sadness, you had to harden your heart. You had to stop being so attached to things and maybe you had to even trick yourself into not caring so much. Maybe you stopped loving as deeply, maybe you stopped believing that you, too, needed help, nurturing, and care.

Sadness is Heart Voice relaying the message: I need comfort. I need help. I have lost something that I valued and I miss it.

### What You Might Be Tempted To Do

You might want to act like you're impervious to such frivolity. You might deem such things as tears, nostalgia, homesickness, and mourning as silly, childish, pointless, or even weak. You might want to think that sadness is no big deal—just par for the course—a mild irritant to be rationalized, overwritten, or justified away. You might be tempted to go for a run, watch a funny movie to distract you, or sweat your ass off in a cycling class. Please don't. Sadness is supposed to be painful. It reminds us of what we loved—sadness is simply the last chapter of that love.

### What Not To Do

In times of despair, lament, and overwhelming sorrow, you might just want to lie down and give up. You might want to curl up in a ball and just stop living altogether. You might want to push people away and wind yourself in barbed wire so that no one ever gets close enough to break your heart again. This might sound reasonable, but it won't help you process your pain, let go of your loss, and heal over. You also might be tempted to just think positive and turn that frown upside down. Sadness isn't something to be glossed over, nor is it something to be talked out of. It is a very human feeling rich with information. Don't skip it. Don't dismiss it. It's there to offer you a clear message—you've lost something that matters.

### What You Should Do

Slow down, put your jammies on, make some tea. Processing sadness is all about cuddling up with cozy comfort. (Remember—babies have it right: cry and then be held.) Ransack your house and bring out all the pillows, blankies, slippers, and soft things you can find. Use these to make yourself a cocoon, a nest, a haven. Call a friend or a loved one to keep you company. If you don't have anyone to call, cuddle up with your pet, or borrow someone else's pet. If you don't have access to a pet, go buy a teddy bear to hug. I'm not kidding. If you honor your sadness (no matter how slight), it clears your heart and allows life-giving emotions to flow freely.

Sadness works like the tides on a seashore. At low tide, everything is raw and exposed. At high tide, the nourishing, life-giving water brings food and resources to rejuvenate the tidal creatures. While everything is raw and exposed, it's best to nest, cocoon, and cozy up. Clearly define exactly what's been lost and what needs to be let go. This means not only naming the love, role, place, or bygone era you've lost—but also the future you'd planned to have.

In ocean-lingo there's a term called slack water—it's the moment in between high and low tides where the water goes slack. There's no movement and for a moment it's standing still. If you watch your sadness carefully, you'll feel this "slack water" within you. You'll notice that suddenly the raw-exposed-nerve-caved-in feeling isn't quite as blinding. This means the tides have changed and now you have to rejuvenate and bring your life force back. Little by little, you regenerate, rejuvenate, revive, and repair.

## On the Mat: Feel Your Emotions

This practice is a meditation on the four core wayfinding emotions. This isn't about trying to artificially create the emotions but rather to allow whatever is within you to surface. Remember: these emotions are not negative, nor are they something to avoid—they offer crucial feedback to help you find your way. Through inquiry, let yourself open to your heart's guidance without judgment. Every time you come to this practice (even within the same day), you may find different answers. Simply allow these answers to arise. By journaling your experience, you'll begin to put words to the wordless. The more time you spend with these feelings, the easier it will be to recognize them, and the more adept you'll become at using your heart for guidance.

*Balancing Pose—Vrksasana*

Stand at the top of your mat. Notice that your body is being held by the ground without you having to think about the solidity of it. Notice that you can count on the ground to be there. Now, let's see what happens when you move into a balancing posture—the pose itself isn't that important as long as you find a way to balance on one foot (without leaning against anything). Bend your right knee to stand on only your left leg. You can simply bend your leg, lifting your foot behind you, or you can wrap your hands around the back of your right thigh—bringing your leg in front of you—while you support your lifted knee. Try to stand on your left leg for two minutes.

While you're balancing, ask yourself: *What am I afraid of?*

Let this be a meditation on fear. Start with the discomfort of the pose. Bring your attention to the feeling of fear within your body. Notice what sensations are related to this feeling. As you begin to wobble and lose your balance, broaden this meditation on fear beyond the pose itself. Notice where you feel this same feeling at home, at work, with your friends, or with your health. See what you can learn about fear while in the safe space of this pose. With full awareness, stand again on both feet and notice any sense of relief, or absence of fear. Journal your insights.

Then repeat this inquiry while balancing on your right leg for two minutes. Take time to notice any difference between sides. Journal your insights.

### Lunge—Anjaneyasana

Come to a standing lunge with your right leg forward. This pose should be difficult, but not impossible. At any time, you can drop your back knee. The intention of this exercise is to create sensation in your hips while opening your heart to shame and guilt. Hold each side for at least two minutes.

On the first side, ask yourself: *What am I ashamed of?*

Let this be a meditation on shame. Start within the pose. Bring your attention to the feeling of shame within your body while you hold the intensity of the lunge. Notice what sensations are related to this feeling. Broaden the meditation beyond the pose itself. Notice where you feel shame throughout your life. See what you can learn about shame while in the safe space of this pose. With full awareness, come out of the pose and notice any sense of relief, or absence of shame. Journal your insights.

Repeat this inquiry by bringing your left leg forward into a lunge. On the second side, bring your inquiry meditation to guilt. Hold for two minutes.

On the second side, ask yourself: *Where do I feel guilty?*

Notice the difference between your experience of shame and your experience of guilt. Start with the pose itself and then broaden your inquiry to where you experience guilt throughout your life. With full awareness, come out of the pose and notice any sense of relief, or absence of guilt. Journal your insights.

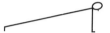

## Plank—Phalakasana

Come to Plank Pose. This pose should be difficult, but not impossible. At any time, you can drop your knees. The intention of this exercise is to create sensation through your core while opening your heart to anger. To hold this pose, you will need to tap into your inner core strength for stability, balance, and power. As your muscles fatigue, you'll be required to dig into a deeper well of strength. As you continue to hold the pose, see if you can shift the focus of strength to muscles surrounding your navel, your core, your back, and your sides. You might get a little wobbly as you hold the pose—notice what muscles help you maintain balance so you can continue to hold yourself outstretched. Hold for at least two minutes.

Ask yourself: *What am I angry about?*

Let this be a meditation on anger. Start within the pose—notice how the pose mirrors the experience of anger in your body. As you continue to hold plank, broaden this meditation on anger beyond the pose itself. Notice where you experience anger in your life. See what you can learn about anger while in the safe space of this pose. With full awareness, come out of the pose, lie down on your belly, and notice any sense of relief, or absence of anger. Journal your insights.

## Open Heart Meditation

Come to a seated cross-legged pose with your spine straight. Extend your arms straight, forming a tall and wide V. Keep your palms flat and facing forward. Close your eyes. Inhale deeply through your nose, and as you exhale hum with your mouth closed. Let the hum resonate through your face, forehead, skull, and upper chest. Continue to hold your arms in an upward stretched V, inhaling through your nose and humming your exhale. Do this for two minutes.

Notice the burning heaviness in your arms and shoulders. This pose should be difficult, but not impossible. At any time, you can drop your arms for a moment, and then return to the pose. The intention of this exercise is to create sensation in your chest while opening your heart to sadness.

Ask yourself: *What do I need to grieve?*

Let this be a meditation on letting go. Start within the pose—notice how the pose mirrors the vulnerable experience of sadness in your body. As you continue to hold your arms, broaden this meditation on sadness beyond the pose itself. Notice where you experience this feeling in the rest of your life. See what you can learn about sadness while in the safe space of this pose. With full awareness, at the two-minute point, keeping your eyes closed, lift your face toward the sky and gently allow your hands to come to your knees, resting palms faceup. Notice the lightness and expansiveness in your chest, head, arms, and shoulders. Notice any sense of relief, or absence of sadness. Journal your insights.

## Off the Mat: Feel Your Emotions

You can check in with the four core wayfinding emotions at any time. By continuing to have a conversation with your Heart Voice, you will become more conscious and aware of the quality of emotion within you. With practice, these feelings become easier to recognize, and the wisdom of each of these emotions will become more accessible to you.

At least once a day, ask yourself:

*What am I afraid of?*

*What am I ashamed of and where do I feel guilty?*

*What am I angry about?*

*What do I need to grieve?*

Record your insights in your journal.

# chapter seven

# When You Can't Handle Your Heart

How to wake up and chart your course
when Heart has taken the wheel.

Your heart is the source from which your emotions flow. When your heart is open and clear, a stream of information flows from it, nourishing your life with the rich intelligence your emotions provide. Each emotion offers you a distinct message and a specific set of directions. But when your heart is blocked and choked, the flow becomes chaotic and unpredictable. The feelings fester and lose their clarity. The emotional water within you becomes muddy and stagnant. In nature, when water stops flowing, the surroundings become dry, brittle, and the ecosystem becomes threatened. Similarly, when your emotions become blocked, your life force can become sick, directionless, and shallow.

In yoga philosophy, these emotional blockages are called *samskara*. Samskara are scars or imprints on your intangible heart. When your heart is open and flowing and feeling every emotion as it comes, everything passes through quickly. Fear runs its course, anger runs its course, sadness runs its course. When your heart is open, as each feeling arises, it's processed in the way that evolution's brilliance intended.

But hearts don't always flow as they should and before you know it, you could find yourself in crisis. Over a lifetime of stress, suffering, and neglect, your heart can become choked down to a mere trickle. Without this crucial force, your mental, emotional, physical, and spiritual well-being becomes critically threatened.

If emotions are essential to our life force, why would we consciously or unconsciously block them? Sometimes, you just don't want to feel every single feeling that comes your way. Sometimes, the emotion is terrible and scary and feels like it might obliterate you, in which case you might close your heart, inwardly turning yourself away from the feeling. Over time, this lessens your capacity to tolerate painful emotions. What was once an open flowing spring becomes a mass of intangible scars choking off your vitality.

## First Thing to Do with a Feeling: Feel It

There are three things you can do with a feeling. The first and most beneficial—but most difficult—is to feel the feeling. That means you allow the rumble, or the pain, or the vibration, or the information, or the message to run through your body. It means you experience the full nature of it—physically. It means you are conscious of the feeling, you can name it—there's an ability to make a discernment about the general nature of it.

By consciously checking in with your Heart Voice and allowing its messages to inform you, you remain the metaphorical driver of your car on the way to your Point B. It means you are connected to the present moment, you're aware of the feedback from the Heart Voice and you're able to navigate using her guidance and direction. You allow the natural life span of the feeling to run its course. You listen to the information and wisdom embedded within the intelligence of the emotion and you take the corresponding action. The spring of your heart runs free and clear, without interference. The emotion runs through you and you respond in real time. This is the way emotions were designed to work, to give you clear information so you could instantly respond and take action. If you're anything like me, you might not really know how to do this feeling-a-feeling thing. Here are a few pointers to help you out:

*Set a time limit for yourself.* Don't attempt to feel all your feelings all at
   once. If you've buried your feelings for a long time, it will take a long

time to get to the source of what you're really feeling. Be patient and set
a timer—fifteen minutes max.

*Stay still and wait*. Distractions keep the feelings at bay. Just stay as still as
you can and quietly wait for whatever arises. Remember that you are the
driver of your car; stay present and listen for feedback without reacting
or turning away.

*Turn inwardly toward your heart and imagine opening it*. The image
that helps for me is a sea anemone in a tide pool when it's open like an
underwater flower. Kids love to poke them and watch them close. Don't
do this to your heart, don't poke it and make it close. Imagine keeping it
loose and open like the sea anemone in high tide.

*It's okay to be afraid*. Fear is a *feeling*, so if you notice you're afraid, you've
already started to *feel*. Congratulations!

*Feelings are like water*. They can be frozen, they can flow, and they can
boil over. Sometimes the hard ones to name have been frozen for a long
time.

*Stop when you can name the feeling*. Don't wallow around in the swamp of
a painful feeling for hours on end. You are new to this practice. Just get
to the point where you can name the emotion, or the greatest part of the
emotion. When the timer goes off, write down any notes in your journal
and go about your regular business.

## Second Thing to Do with a Feeling: Avoid It

The second and very common option is to avoid feeling your feelings. This
option is an inner turning-away from pain—deliberately or unconsciously.
Instead of remaining in the driver's seat, you disconnect from the present
moment and jump into the backseat of your life.

This avoidance of the Heart Voice could be a deliberate pushing away,
stuffing, disregarding, or compartmentalizing of emotion. Maybe you don't
want to cry during a fight, so you suck in your sadness and muscle yourself through the conversation without allowing yourself to feel the sadness
and loss. Maybe you avoid having the conversation in the first place, and
instead avoid phone calls and texts—hoping it will all go away. Maybe you

don't want to show weakness, so you cough or clear your throat rather than allow your voice to betray your sense of vulnerability.

Avoiding your feelings might also show up as an unconscious turning away—most often toward distraction or self-soothing. It could be as small as picking up your phone to avoid feeling bored. It could be madly cleaning your house to avoid a feeling of powerlessness. It could be bingeing on Net-flix to avoid a feeling of loneliness. Instead of stuffing, ignoring, or burying the feeling, you run away from your feelings and throw yourself into any-thing that brings a little relief.

When you're avoiding your feelings, you're not experiencing them as evolution intended. You're not driving your life any longer. When you re-press your emotions, Heart is now unconsciously running the show. She's at the wheel when you push pause and have a margarita. She's at the wheel when you put your feelings into a box while you go for a run. She's at the wheel when you file away your feelings for a rainy day while keeping busy at the office.

The problem with this is that the more you run from your feelings, the more there are to run from. The more you avoid, the more there is to avoid. Emotions don't disappear when you ignore them, they merely fester and wreak havoc behind the scenes. When you avoid a feeling, you're merely procrastinating. The feeling will wait. And while it waits, it will get bigger, uglier, more complicated, and more confusing.

As the pain and discomfort increases, the intensity of the avoidance tac-tic must also increase. The greater the pain, the more intensity you need to distract yourself from it. What starts off as a seemingly benign habit can grow into a life-shattering addiction. Whether you are drinking, eat-ing, starving, spending, gambling, snorting, sniffing, smoking, running, or *anything-else*-ing, when you continue a behavior despite the negative con-sequences that it creates in your life, it means—at its root—that you're in pain.

Show me someone who can't stop punishing themselves, someone who can't put their phone down, their drink down, their laptop down, someone who can't just be here in this moment without having to alter it or self-soothe through it—and I'll show you someone who doesn't know how to handle their Heart Voice. I'll show you someone who has made a habit of disconnecting and jumping into the backseat of her life. When you have inwardly turned away so often that your feelings have become overwhelming mountains towering over you, they seem to threaten you with utter annihilation. So, you up the ante. You drink more. You eat more. You purge more. You work more. You fill-in-the-blank more—desperately trying to self-soothe, grasping for any sense of relief as the unprocessed feelings loom with doom. It's a painful cycle that can only be ended one way: learning to listen to your heart's guidance.

## Clearing the Heart

If your heart has become blocked and impeded, you'll have to work very hard to clear the clutter and debris. If you have a month, year—lifetime?— of unprocessed painful feelings, you may have quite a chore in front of you. Ideally, you should just be able to flip your heart switch to the "on" position and then go on your merry way. But life doesn't work like that and neither does your heart. For every unprocessed moment, for every time you closed your heart, for every time you ate a Snickers bar or drank a martini, or mindlessly scrolled through Facebook to avoid a feeling, the unprocessed moment now waits for you.

I'm not saying that now you're sentenced to a lifetime of emotional-suffering, nor am I saying that you can't clear through the muck to free your heart. I'm just saying it will be a slow process of clawing your way through the intangible blockages. If your mom died when you were little and you have a bunch of stuck grief, it means you start digging through the grief, naming it, and taking the corresponding action (sadness means to let go and rejuvenate). If you got divorced six years ago and merely soldiered through it with a stiff upper lip, it means you might start ripping through grief, and anger, and fear, and shame. It means bit by bit you start to dig through the old stuff and feel each feeling enough to be able to name it and work through it.

This is not a small task, it's probably the work of your life. But day by day, the heart starts to flow easier and more clearly. As this life force starts to flow through you, you'll become more adept at feeling your feelings and using their feedback for guidance.

## Third Thing to Do with a Feeling: Support It

So, let's be honest. Sometimes you just don't want to feel a feeling. I mean, joy and happiness and excitement are great but who really wants to sign up for anger, sadness, shame, and fear? They are inconvenient. They aren't fun; in fact, they can be really uncomfortable.

When you first fall in love, you want that feeling to last forever but it doesn't; that sky-high feeling fades into a quieter, and often deeper, connection. The same is true of painful feelings—even the worst grief will fade. Allowing the full experience of an emotion—like it or not—is essential if you want to use your heart for guidance. If you give yourself a time limit, an expiration date, and clear parameters, you could probably feel just about anything. If you had to feel intense grief for twenty-seven days and five hours, you could. If you were subjected to feeling hot, burning shame for twelve minutes, you could. Or, rage. You wouldn't necessarily *want* to feel any of those extreme emotions, but you *could*. Your heart was designed to bear and carry so much more than you believe you can.

If only our most painful experiences and emotions could be prepared for. But life doesn't work like this. It's not predictable. It's not safe. It's not controllable. There's no clear-cut schedule to any of this. There's no way to know how long or how intensely you're ever going to have to feel. There's no way to know how long you'll have to endure something difficult.

The natural life span of a feeling is just a few moments. But what if the scary thing keeps happening? What if the perpetrator keeps hunting you? What if the exile doesn't let up? What if the boundary violator keeps coming at you? What if you lose one thing and then another and then another and the sadness just doesn't let up? What if the attacker hasn't attacked yet, but you know that he's just waiting for the right time?

Even though an emotion may run its course, a new bit of information can trigger a cycle of emotion. This can create immense amounts of suffering and can easily send you into an emotional spiral. The Heart Voice is incredibly important to listen to—you need its guidance. But you also need to temper this with kindness and compassion for yourself.

When times get difficult and you feel a prolonged sense of discomfort or suffering, or there is no action that can be taken in the present moment—instead of an unconscious distraction—you can deliberately choose to support yourself through the difficult feeling. The art of wayfinding isn't about becoming some sort of spiritual athlete and the goal here isn't to brave through raw open-nerve-suffering, but rather to find a way to support the Heart Voice so that it can continue to offer clear guidance. By using tools, props, and purposeful distractions, you can help yourself through any difficult challenge.

The Yoga Sutra of Patanjali 2.46 states, "Asana is a steady, comfortable posture."[9] Originally written in Sanskrit, the language of ancient India, as "sthira sukhamasanam." *Asanam* means yoga pose or posture, *sthira* means steady and stable, and *sukha* means comfortable, ease, and pleasant. This sutra teaches that a yoga pose should be steady and stable while abiding in ease and comfort. The sutra *does not* teach that the pose should make you grunt, or sweat, or pull a muscle, give yourself a hernia, grit your teeth, or lose your breath. The posture or pose is meant to be steady and comfortable. Many teachers will guide you to find your *edge* in a pose. This edge is a place where you can abide comfortably while staying connected to your breath. The minute you're huffing and puffing and pulling and scraping your way into a pose (or out of one), you've lost the nature or essence of the pose and you've gone past your edge.

For some of us, the idea of putting your ankles behind your head, doing full lotus, or even comfortably sitting cross-legged might be way beyond what our bodies are capable of doing—let alone trying to get in or out of any of these poses with steadiness and ease. Even common poses such as Child's Pose, Forward Fold, or Pigeon might be a far cry from reality for many. For this reason, most yoga studios have props to help support you so you can learn to hold the pose with steadiness and ease. Instead of forcing your body to do something it can't, or completely skipping any pose

---

9. Satchidananda, *The Yoga Sutra of Patanjali*, 142.

beyond your physical level of flexibility or strength, you can use a prop to keep you in position.

I used to rebuff any prop suggestion in class. I'd snub the idea of needing help or assistance and saw props as "cheating." I'd also grip and sweat and hold my breath and force my body into shapes it wasn't ready for and for way longer than anything that resembled steadiness or ease. And I got injured. A lot. I sprained my toe. I broke my wrist. I hurt my back more times than I can count. And once, I accidentally fell right on top of my head, tweaking my neck so badly that I couldn't turn my head for a week.

This is not unlike how I tried to cope with my Heart Voice. For years I thought I was just supposed to suck it up and grind my way through emotional suffering. I was militant in not allowing myself grace, ease, or support. I saw spirituality as an emotional competition—the winner being the one to endure the most pain. I wanted to be good and I wanted to do it right. I didn't want to cheat. So I stayed strong and carried on and ended up emotionally bruised and battered to the point where I was forced to try a different strategy.

After decades of injuries, I finally surrendered and began using props in my yoga practice. Once I embraced using props, my practice deepened, my body relaxed, and I could feel—day by day—that my body was learning to trust me in a different way. I could find the *edge* of the pose and hold it with steadiness and with ease. I allowed myself time to provide props for myself and relished in the abundance of having as much support as possible. My practice began to nourish me and replenish me rather than injure me and deplete me.

As I learned this skill on the mat, I began to connect ways to use "props" off the mat. As I learned how to bolster and support my body so that I could hold a difficult pose with abiding steadiness and ease, I learned that I could bolster and support a difficult life event so that I could keep my heart open with abiding steadiness and ease.

## On the Mat: Prop on Purpose

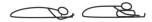

*Seated Forward Fold with and without Props—Paschimottanasana*

If you own yoga props, gather two bolsters and a blanket. If you do not own yoga bolsters—two bath towels, a blanket (throw size), and a few pillows will work just fine. Keep your pen and journal nearby.

First, try a Seated Forward Fold without any props. See if you can abide in this pose with steadiness and ease. Notice if the backs of your legs begin to hurt or if your neck or back start to strain. If so, you've gone too far. Bring yourself out of the pose until you find a comfortable edge.

Hold this unsupported forward fold for three minutes.

While in the pose, ask yourself: *What thoughts, feelings, or physical sensations come up in this unsupported pose? Where in my life am I trying to hold a difficult edge? What is the emotional quality of this edge in my life? Where in my life am I struggling to find steadiness and ease?*

Take a moment to journal your insights.

Next, do the same shape or pose with your body, but this time offer yourself as much support as possible. As an experiment, allow yourself to go overboard and use extreme self-care in the pose. The goal of using props isn't to change the pose, it's to allow your body to be able to be in pose with steadiness and ease. That way, you're able to garner all the benefits of the pose without any stress.

To fully experience this pose, have your legs straight out in front of you and lay a pillow or bolster lengthwise on top of your legs. If you're super flexible, you can do this with straight legs and just lay your torso down over your thighs without the pillow support. If it's too much, roll a blanket (or two towels together) and place them under your knees for support. You might also need to lift your pelvis to allow your hips to fold forward. If so, you can fold a blanket and place it under your tailbone, helping to tip your pelvis forward. You might also place a pillow (or two or three) on top of your legs so your torso can relax onto the support. The idea is to bring the floor up to your body, to bolster your body so you can allow your weight to sink into the pose. Even if you're heavily propped, your legs are still generally out in front of you and your torso is generally lying forward over them. By using props, you allow yourself the benefits of the posture. Hold your supported forward fold for three minutes.

While in the pose, ask yourself: *How does the experience of the supported pose compare to the unsupported pose? What thoughts, feelings, or physical sensations come up in the supported pose? What "pose" (difficult situation) is life asking of me right now? How can I "prop this pose" (offer support that creates a positive consequence) to help me find steadiness and ease?*

Take a moment to journal your insights.

## Off the Mat: Prop on Purpose

Now let's take your on-the-mat insights into the rest of your life. I find it helpful to look at difficult situations or emotions as metaphorical yoga poses. You might not be ready for full frontal contact with your Heart Voice. And that's okay! There are no awards given out for pain endurance. But you can always choose to support yourself with kindness.

### Props for Fear

Fear is a high intensity, very vibrate-y feeling. Props for fear also need to be high intensity and probably need to include movement, intense creativity, hard work, extreme focus, or manual labor (something that makes you sweat). If you're going through a particularly fearful time, you might want to offer yourself support to get yourself through it.

Things that I've found to help fear:

- *True crime and mystery—books, podcasts, TV shows, and movies.* It might sound odd that reading or watching scary things might help support you through a scary time, but trust me—this works. Something about having a specific and focused fear allows your insides to settle down. Rather than just being overwhelmed by your vague out-there-all-around fear, channeling it into a thrilling detective mystery seems to help the nervous system weirdly relax—as if it now has something to focus on.

- *High intensity exercise.* Hike, run, dance, jump, shake, bounce—do something to the point of exhaustion. The fear response is: Run—so help your body do what it's programmed to do—move.
- *Making something from scratch.* Fear is about not having control. It's helpless and powerless. It's about not being able to predict something. So, make something, anything. Write a book, paint a picture, bake a cake, knit a scarf, build a bench, paint a dresser. Do something that gives you some sense of being able to influence an outcome.
- *Doing something difficult.* Dig a ditch. Chop wood. Carry buckets of water. Rake the leaves. Weed the garden. Do something that requires sweat and even blood or tears. This helps you strengthen your body giving yourself a signal that you're ready and able to run.
- *Swaddling and physical compression.* If you don't have a weighted blanket, you can swaddle yourself (yes, as in what you do to babies— don't knock it 'till you try it). Basically, you take a blanket and wrap it around you as tightly as possible. The compression helps to alleviate the physical symptoms of fear. If you like this feeling, you can get yourself a weighted blanket. I rely on my weighted blanket to ground me—it's my favorite go-to for fear, anxiety, worry, uncertainty, and doubt. You can find these online listed as trauma blankets, gravity blankets, or weighted blankets. It instantly comforts me and helps me feel safe. The compression keeps me connected to my current surroundings and helps me feel protected in the moment.

### Props for Shame and Guilt

Shame and guilt tend to make us want to hide, keep secrets, isolate, and stay away from the group. But the Heart Voice message behind shame and guilt is to connect with others. Therefore, props for shame and guilt are to help us connect in tiny and manageable ways. If you're going through a particularly shame-y and guilt-ridden time, you might want to offer yourself support to get yourself through it.

Things that I've found to help shame and guilt:

- *Feed someone.* Bake some cookies, make a casserole, put some bread in a basket. Back in the olden days, we'd feed each other as a way to connect. We'd offer neighbors, friends, and family food. This isn't so much about the eating as it is about the making of something to give to someone else. Shame is a very self-conscious and self-absorbed feeling. This prop is about moving the focus to others—ideally someone who might also need connection.

- *Put some lipstick on.* Or a cute outfit. Or just freaking brush your hair. Do something that signals (to yourself) that you care. A little bit of effort goes a long way when you're in a shame spiral. Do not sequester yourself to sweatpants, ratty sweaters, and worn-out slippers. Even if you don't feel like it, make yourself put on something that reinforces that you are worthy of care and attention.

- *Hang out with an animal.* If you don't have a pet, find access to one. You can go to a local shelter or to a pet store or even go to your local dog park and just simply watch the dogs play. If you're feeling really shame-y and like you want to crawl up in a hole and die, animals can be a way to help you feel connected.

- *Be with people.* Go to a meeting, a yoga class, to church, to a meditation group. Join a meet-up. Go to a museum. Sit on a bench in the middle of a park, or a mall, or near a well-traveled trail. Get yourself off the couch and put yourself in a place with other people. You don't have to make friends with the people, but just put yourself back among humans—trust me, it helps.

- *Cover your mirrors.* Pretend you're a vampire and stay away from mirrors. Turn them around or put a towel or sheet over them for a while. If you're like me, when you're in a shame spiral you can lose minutes (years!) berating yourself in the mirror. It's incredible how quickly you start to feel better when you're not spending so much time obsessing about your image.

*Props for Anger*

Anger is similar to fear in that it's high intensity and to prop it, you'll need to use something as intense. The Heart Voice message behind anger is: Fight and protect! Therefore, props for anger are to help you maintain your inner strength so you're ready to fight when needed. If you're going through a particularly angry time, you might want to offer yourself support to get yourself through it.

Things that I've found to help anger:

- *Watch an action flick.* A good hero saga or underdog-turned-hero story—same as crime and mystery for fear, watching healthy anger in action helps to alleviate the internal turbulence. Action movies or a good under-dog prevailing movie helps you to feel your own anger while being inspired by the story's strength and the hero's courage.

- *Scream into your pillow.* Find a fluffy pillow (or you'll scare the neighbors) and howl as loudly as you can into it. Use profanity. Spew hate or just scream bloody murder. Do this for a few minutes, until your core muscles and your vocal chords are tired. This can end up being quite silly—don't take yourself too seriously here. (Kids love this one!) Just channel the anger through your voice. Repeat as often as necessary.

- *Use your muscles.* Anger prepares the body for fight—so use the strength and work out. Run stairs. Lift heavy objects. Jump rope. Do sit-ups. Pump iron. (Think: Rocky.) Work the anger through your body.

- *Sing.* Anger wants you to set boundaries, speak up and use your voice. If you're in a stuck anger pattern (where you can't take action yet), use your voice in a different way: sing. The louder the better. Turn on a good anthem and sing in the shower, or in the car, or somewhere where you won't be tempted to temper your volume.

- *Get rid of shit.* Even seeing that sentence makes my blood temperature rise and brings a wicked smile to my face. When I'm having to relentlessly work through anger, there's nothing like going through old shit and making piles to take to the dump or to Goodwill. The internal need to set a boundary, to move things away from me, and to attack the bad guy all gets funneled into clearing out clutter and getting rid of burdensome crap.

### Props for Sadness

Sadness is a slow-moving, lingering feeling that comes in and out like waves. To prop it, you'll need to use something soothing, slow, and patient. The Heart Voice message behind sadness is: Let go and rejuvenate. Therefore, props for sadness are to help comfort you through the letting-go process. If you're going through a particularly broken-hearted time, gentle props can help support you as you navigate the waves of sadness.

Things that I've found to help sadness:

- *Read a book.* Reading requires you to slow down and be in the quiet; its pace is slow and matches sadness well. A book can take you both outside the venue of your own pain, and into other worlds. The newness of a novel, or the complex narrative of a time in history, or even a business book, can connect you to others in a gentle and anonymous way, at a time when we feel the hollow of sadness, a time when we might be tempted to disconnect and retreat. A book can help prepare our heart to both grieve openly, and also to fill back up with all the love and mystery of living that waits for us just on the other side of that sadness. Sadness says something you love is gone. Books remind us of beginnings.

- *Watch a sad (but not too sad) movie.* Watch a movie that helps you open your heart and see the beauty in humanity. Watch a movie like *Cast Away, Lars and the Real Girl,* or *Love Actually*—tear-jerkers with sweetness. Stay away from anything that's too doom and gloom, depressing, or tragic.

- *Listen to your favorite music—the sadder the better.* Some of the best songs ever written were created to help the songwriter process heartbreak, hurt, and sadness. Listening to someone else sing about what you're feeling can be immensely relieving. Music helps to evoke the beauty of this rich emotion and helps you slowly let go.

- *Wear soft clothes.* I spoke about making a nest or haven for sadness in chapter 7, and this is taking it one step further—to wearing a "nest." Sadness wants softness, it wants fluffy, flexible, cottony, cushiony comfort. To support sadness, refuse to wear anything confining, rough or tough. Instead, reach for jersey, cashmere, or the softest fleece you can find.

- *Get in water.* Sadness comes in waves. It works like the tides, taking out the old and bringing in the new. When you're going through a particularly sad time, put your body into water. Find a hot spring, a local mineral bath, a hot tub, the ocean itself, or a pool. Soak, float, swim. Allow your body to be held and buoyed by the water.

- *Be in nature.* Find a trail or a park or a beach or a river or somewhere that's as close to nature as possible. Notice the trees, plants, and wildlife. Notice the rocks and the earth and the contours of the landscape. Feel the heat of the sun on your face. Feel each step you take and notice how the earth supports you. You are not alone in this process of letting go. Everything lives and everything dies in nature. The sun rises and the sun sets again. By being in nature, you connect to the order of things and can support yourself and allow the exquisite pain of letting go.

part two closing

# Wayfinding with Your Heart Voice

You can use the wisdom of your Heart Voice through the practice of inquiry. Inquiry helps you to clarify Heart's message, and to determine the advice or direction that the voice offers you. Heart's messages are sometimes wrapped in very strong emotions, but the Heart Voice is never petty or irrelevant.

The Heart Voice speaks through emotions, which give you clear feedback and direct you to take particular actions. Through inquiry, you will take each of the core wayfinding emotions into consideration so you can clarify Heart's message and find the emotional truth of the situation. To find your way, stay present while you feel your feelings, become conscious of any habits you use to avoid your feelings, and learn to trust your heart for guidance. Although certain emotions might be more dominant, they do not stand alone. In every situation, you should consider each of the core wayfinding emotions: fear, shame/guilt, anger, and sadness. Even if you're not consciously aware of these feelings, through inquiry you may find that they offer even deeper wisdom than what might be noticeable on the surface.

# Heart Inquiry Method

*What's the situation?*

Whether you want to clarify a difficult situation, get to your version of Point B, make a decision, or find your way when you're entirely lost—start with articulating your situation. In just a sentence or two, write a short version of your dilemma, quandary, or story.

*What emotion(s) come up for you in this situation? How do you feel?*

If you're not sure, look through the list of feelings within each of the core mapmaking groups to help you determine which feelings are most dominant.

- **Fear Family—the emotional response to danger:** alert, apprehensive, cautious, concerned, confused, disoriented, disquieted, doubtful, bored, edgy, fidgety, hesitant, indecisive, insecure, unsure, pensive, shy, timid, uneasy, watchful, angst, afraid, on guard, anxious, scared, fearful, helpless, jumpy, nervous, rattled, restless, stressed, startled, suspicious, unsettled, wary, worried, filled with dread, overwhelmed, horrified, panicked, paralyzed, petrified, phobic, shocked, terrorized, mistrustful, vigilant, vulnerable, trepidatious

- **Shame and Guilt Family—the emotional response to possible social disconnection:** awkward, flustered, hesitant, withdrawn, self-conscious, ashamed, chagrined, contrite, culpable, embarrassed, feeling worthless, guilty, humbled, intimidated, penitent, regretful, remorseful, sheepish, belittled, degraded, demeaned, disgraced, less than, humiliated, mortified, ostracized, self-loathing, marginalized, stigmatized, inauthentic, fraudulent, incapable, disingenuous, sensitive, exposed, unfaithful, on the spot, out on a limb, revealing, self-conscious, tender, thin-skinned, weak, defenseless, naked, powerless, unsafe, unguarded, not-enough, damaged, unwanted, rejected, regret, remorse, wide open, unworthy, unloved, broken, banished, exiled, mortified, dishonored, insecure, repentant, shy, sorry, submissive, grandiose, vulnerable to loss of connection

- **Anger Family—the emotional response to boundary violation and unfairness:** annoyed, apathetic, bitter, bored, certain, cold, crabby, cranky, critical, cross, detached, displeased, frustrated, impatient, indif-

ferent, irritated, peeved, rankled, affronted, aggravated, angry, antago-
nized, arrogant, bristling, exasperated, incensed, indignant, inflamed,
mad, offended, resentful, riled up, sarcastic, aggressive, appalled, bel-
ligerent, bitter, contemptuous, disgusted, furious, hateful, hostile, irate,
livid, menacing, outraged, rage, ranting, raving, seething, spiteful,
vengeful, vicious, vindictive, violent, jealous, envious, hateful, malice,
ill will, grudging, malevolent, malicious, spiteful, intolerant, protective,
possessive, skeptical, taken advantage of, abused, mistreated, bullied,
shamed, lied to, determined, protective, on guard

- **Sadness Family—the emotional response to loss:** contemplative, blue,
down in the dumps, disappointed, disconnected, discouraged, distracted,
grounded, hurt feelings, listless, low, nostalgic, melancholy, regretful,
heartsick, steady, wistful, crushed, dejected, discouraged, dispirited,
down, downtrodden, drained, forlorn, gloomy, grieving, heavy-hearted,
melancholy, mournful, sad, sorrowful, weepy, world-weary, anguished,
bereaved, bleak, depressed, despairing, despondent, betrayed, devastated,
grief-stricken, heartbroken, hopeless, inconsolable, morose, homesick,
dark, miserable, poignant, tragic, unhappy, upset, sentimental, wistful,
lonesome, longing, yearning, loss, disconnection

### *Are you afraid of anything here? If so, why? What is the specific danger? What action needs to be taken to keep you safe?*

Healthy fear hones your senses, alerts your innate survival skills, and increases your ability to respond effectively to changing environments. Fear
is an alert to get you to flee from danger. Name the reality-based specific
danger, the nature of the actual threat to your real life. You might notice
you have a slew of imaginary threats that aren't concrete real-life scenarios.
This might show up as a general feeling of powerlessness, where nothing
feels predictable or safe. You might notice a strong desire to gain control
over people, places, events, the future, or the universe at large. This is what
happens when your Heart Voice reacts to your Mind Voice.

To calm these Mind-based fears, use Mind Voice tools. Fear is about
running from danger—it's the "flight" in your fight-or-flight response. It
wants you to get away from the Bad Guy. It wants you to remove yourself

from the danger. (If you get really stuck here, you might need to work the Mind Voice tools first to clear out the chatter.) Once you've specified the danger, list what actions can be taken to help keep you safe. List specific things you can do to protect yourself from the danger present in this situation.

### *Are you feeling guilty and/or ashamed about anything here? If so, why? What social hierarchy, status, bond, or relationship is being threatened? How can you restore your sense of belonging and connection?*

Shame and guilt show up when a relationship or social connection is threatened and trigger an early warning sign to help you stop behaving in a way that would lead to ostracism, exclusion, banishment, or exile. Consider who or what has been wronged in this situation, what relationship has been threatened, or if your social hierarchy might be damaged. Specify what actions need to be taken to repair the relationship, or to move toward intimacy and vulnerability with someone you trust. This might mean saying you're sorry, making amends, repairing damage, and owning your part. It also might mean connecting with someone who has nothing to do with this situation and taking the risk to allow yourself to be seen, understood, and witnessed.

### *Are you angry about anything here? If so, why? What needs to be protected? What needs to be communicated?*

Anger shows up to keep you (and your loved ones) safe. It shows up as a response to any situation where your goal is being thwarted or stymied. Whether someone (or something) has violated your boundary, or something has become increasingly unfair—anger ensures that you fight, hold your ground, and protect what's yours. Boundaries are guidelines—tangible or intangible limits—that help to clearly define what needs to be protected. Anger signals that a boundary has been violated and asks for you to protect where the breech occurred. Boundaries are rules or limits you set for how people behave and interact with you and yours. They are also specific personal guidelines for what happens when someone crosses those limits. Clarify what boundary has been breached and what course of action is necessary for you to restore your boundary.

Healthy boundaries are a critical part of creating honest relationships and connections that thrive. In yoga, we practice movement and meditation in community but we also learn how to stay on our own mat. The best teachers may offer props or adjustments, but their guidance should be gentle and they should honor each student's willingness or unwillingness to accept touch or direction. Yoga is communal but it is also deeply personal. All of our relationships are this way: there is a deep need for connection, and there are the limits and boundaries that each individual chooses. The practice of setting boundaries can be quite complicated. I'd love to dive head first into this subject, but boundary work is vast and really merits an entire book on the subject—so I'll just give you an overview of how boundaries work.

- Boundaries are not complaints, threats, or ultimatums. They aren't mean, cruel, or rude. They are your rules for who, what, how, and why you feel comfortable being closer to someone else—clear communication of what's true for you—helping others know who you are and how to interact with you. A boundary can be a firm line in the sand, or a very subtle shift. When we are clear with our boundaries, no one who meets us, works with us, or tries to emotionally connect with us is left guessing.

- Boundaries are not about trying to make someone else change. Instead, you state your request and wait. Sometimes you're lucky and the person hears your request and honors it immediately. But if you've been a bit of a noodle-y-people-pleasing-doormat, you might be up to your eyeballs in boundary violators. If so, *you* will probably have to be the one to take the necessary action to protect and restore your boundary. For example, instead of complaining that someone keeps calling too late, you'd communicate, "I turn my phone off after 8:00 p.m." Instead of policing their behavior, you'd simply turn your phone to do-not-disturb so you're not bothered. You change your behavior to create the boundary rather than wait for the other person to honor your request.

• When you're trying to set clear boundaries, a simple *yes* or *no, thank you* works wonders. When someone does something that breeches your boundary, say something like, "That doesn't work for me," or "That doesn't feel good to me." If someone repeatedly tries to contact you, you can say, "Please do not call/text/email/show up again." If (when) they do it again, unfollow, unfriend, block their phone number, their social media access to you, or set up an email filter to protect your valuable space, time, and energy.

• When someone violates a boundary, you start by clearly stating your request. A request focuses on what you want rather than putting the focus on what you don't want. A possible request script is: "I would like _____" Or: "I would appreciate _____." (Keep it very simple. The fewer words the better.)

• The person may or may not honor your request. No matter what course of action the person takes, their behavior is crucial feedback. If they honor your request, it will likely create calm within the relationship, a sense of equality and balance. If they ignore your request, you can take the necessary actions to protect and restore your boundary. Remove yourself from a situation, leave the party, shut a door, hang up, do what's needed to create the boundary yourself.

• Boundaries are even more important when we want to stay in a relationship, a friendship, a working partnership—to allow a relationship to grow with the understanding that each person within that relationship deserves to set their own limits, to ask clearly for what they want and do not want. Healthy boundaries bring us all closer to people we feel ready to trust, people who see us, respect us, and choose repeatedly to respect the boundaries that keep us safe, and keep our sense of selves intact.

*Are you sad? If so, why? What has been lost? What must be revived?*

Sadness comes up when you lose something of value. It helps you slow down, feel your losses, and let go of that which needs to be released—to soften into the flow of life instead of holding yourself rigidly and pushing onward. Specify what's been lost, even if it's an imaginary idea. The more specific the better. To help the tides of sadness move through, also consider what must be revived. For any loss, there's a call for rejuvenation and res-toration. With any death, there's a rebirth that wants to take its place. All emotions have different intensities, importance, and duration depending on the situation but certain kinds of sadness—deep grief, sustained pain, or betrayal—aren't quick fixes. Deeper wounds require focused recognition of the need to let go, and support to allow that letting go to happen in the most gentle way possible. If you try to speed up real grief, you will fail. You simply have to give bigger experiences and very strong emotions the room they need.

*Which feelings are the most dominant in this situation?*
*What guidance is Heart offering?*

Fear's advice is: Stay safe! Shame and guilt's advice is: Connect with some-one! Anger's advice is: Protect your boundaries! Sadness's advice is: Let go. Determine which feelings are dominant in this situation so you can clarify Heart's guidance.

*Specify your Point B for this particular situation.*

Think about the big picture and articulate your larger intention, focus, commitment, and priority.

*Is Heart's advice taking you to where you want to go?*

Considering your Point B, decide if Heart's advice will get you where you really want to go.

*To help you stay connected to your heart in this situation, what "prop" or support might help you hold this "pose" with steadiness and ease?*
You might not be ready to fully embrace the emotion offered by your Heart Voice. Choose an activity that helps support you through this difficult situation without creating negative consequences for yourself.

*Thank Heart and move her to the backseat.*
Here's your new script: "Thank you, Heart, for trying to help me _____. I won't always be able to take your advice, but I truly appreciate your input. My larger intention, focus, commitment, and priority is _____. I will stay connected to your wisdom as I move in that direction."

## Quick Review of the Heart Inquiry Method

1. What's the situation?
2. What emotion(s) come up for you in this situation? How do you feel?
3. Are you afraid of anything here? If so, why? What is the specific danger? What action needs to be taken to keep you safe?
4. Are you feeling guilty and/or ashamed about anything here? If so, why? What social hierarchy, status, bond, or relationship is being threatened? How can you restore your sense of belonging and connection?
5. Are you angry about anything here? If so, why? What needs to be protected? What needs to be communicated?
6. Are you sad? If so, why? What has been lost? What must be revived?
7. Which feelings are the most dominant in this situation? What guidance is Heart offering?
8. Specify your Point B for this particular situation.
9. Is Heart's advice taking you to where you want to go?
10. To help you stay connected to your heart in this situation, what "prop" or support might help you hold this "pose" with steadiness and ease?

11. Thank Heart and move her to the backseat. Here's your new script: "Thank you, Heart, for trying to help me _____. I won't always be able to take your advice, but I truly appreciate your input. My larger intention, focus, commitment, and priority is _____. I will stay connected to your wisdom as I move in that direction."

### Example: A Friendship Issue

1. **What's the situation?** My sister doesn't seem concerned with what's happening in my life. I had a major win to celebrate and didn't hear back from her for days. When I did hear back, I got a couple of emojis via text. It felt like a slap in the face, like I didn't matter.

2. **What emotion(s) come up for you in this situation? How do you feel?** I feel really frustrated and disrespected. I feel like I'm worth more than this. I am tired of being patient. I do not deserve this. I feel like I've lost my sister and that this has progressively gotten worse over the past few years. Dominant emotions are anger and sadness.

3. **Are you afraid of anything here? If so, why? What is the specific danger? What action needs to be taken to keep you safe?** I am afraid that I'm losing her. I'm also afraid to share myself with her. It feels unsafe. The specific danger seems to be if I share my intimate thoughts and feelings, or things that deeply matter to me, she will respond with boredom or a dull sense of obligation. Until I feel a sense of reciprocity, the action would be to be more careful about what I share and what I expect from the relationship.

4. **Are you feeling guilty and/or ashamed about anything here? If so, why? What social hierarchy, status, bond, or relationship is being threatened? How can you restore your sense of belonging and connection?** I have checked myself over and over to see if I have behaved poorly, or if I've not been there for her. I keep wondering if this is some sort of passive aggressive payback for something that I may have missed. I can't find any wrongdoing here—no guilt. This

definitely plays into my "not good enough, don't matter, not important" feelings though. So, it feels like there's a level of shame underneath all of this. I think our friendship is being threatened—or at least the friendship that we once had is threatened. I can restore my sense of belonging and connection by purposely reaching out and sharing this pain with someone I trust. Someone who feels safe.

5. **Are you angry about anything here? If so, why? What needs to be protected? What needs to be communicated?** I'm tired of reaching out and being ignored. I need to set a boundary with myself. It's been clear for over a year that she's not available in the way that she used to be and not capable or interested in the same level of intimacy. Heart is saying: protect yourself, step away from this. I don't know that I need to communicate this boundary to anyone except myself.

6. **Are you sad? If so, why? What has been lost? What must be revived?** I am sad because I have lost a very valuable part of my life. I keep trying to reach out, but she's not mutually reaching back. I need to let go of the old relationship so that I can accept the one that we now have. Rather than expecting her to be by my side for all things, I can still love her for who she is *now* in my life. I also can admit that my real needs are not being met by this particular friendship, and acknowledge that I do want to have deep and meaningful relationships—to revive, I need to invest in other friendships.

7. **Which feelings are the most dominant in this situation? What guidance is Heart offering?** Anger and sadness. Protect my boundaries and let go. Honor her boundaries—even if her boundaries feel murky and unclear—and let go.

8. **Specify your Point B for this particular situation.** To have meaningful and intimate friendships in my life.

9. **Is Heart's advice taking you to where you want to go?** Yes, if I stop trying to hold on to something that's no longer there, I can focus on moving toward building and strengthening other relationships.

10. **To help you stay connected to your heart in this situation, what "prop" or support might help you hold this "pose" with steadiness and ease?** I can talk through this with someone I love and trust. I can reach out to start to strengthen other relationships. I can spend more time on the relationships in my life that feel reciprocal.

11. **Thank Heart and move her to the backseat.** Here's your new script: "Thank you, Heart, for trying to help me protect and let go. I won't always be able to take your advice, but I truly appreciate your input. My larger intention, focus, commitment, and priority is to have meaningful friendships in my life. I will stay connected to your wisdom as I move in that direction."

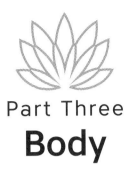

## Part Three
# Body

The body's voice communicates through the animal of your human body. Its voice is driven by instinct and has evolved over eons to help keep you alive and thriving. As we move forward through the next few chapters, you'll learn basic tools to help you listen and respond to the voice of your body. I'll show you what happens when you check out and let Body drive your life, and I'll teach you how you can access your inner body wisdom through inquiry.

chapter eight

# The Body Voice

An introduction to the voice of the body.
How it works, how to recognize it,
and how it influences your journey.

Your body is an animal. The Body Voice is the voice of that animal, the information that comes not only from the tangible part of your body—through pain, pleasure, sensations, hunger, thirst, energy, exhaustion—but also the information that comes through the instinctual, intangible wisdom that has evolved over eons to help you survive.

To be able to survive, your body needs to be able to tell you if it's in danger. Just like your hand pulls itself away from a hot flame, your body instinctually wants to preserve itself. It wants to stay alive. It communicates its various needs through physical sensations—sometimes subtle (think: dry mouth, tired eyes, hunger pangs) and sometimes intense (think: labor pains, vertigo, traveler's diarrhea). Your body will tell you when it needs food, water, rest, protection, touch, or shelter. Sensations such as hunger, thirst, hot, cold, pain, and pleasure communicate the Body Voice easily if you're aware, present, and listening. The animal of your body offers cues such as hunger and thirst to help you know when it needs nourishment. It offers cues such as sleepiness or fatigue to help you know that it needs rest. It offers pleasure and comfort to help you know that it craves touch and connection.

The animal of your body needs to know where it is in the world—your actual location in comparison to what it might need. It becomes frightened or stressed when it doesn't know how, when, or where food, water, shelter, or safety will be obtained. It becomes frightened or stressed if it doesn't know how to get home. Humans survive and thrive with social support, so your body also knows that it needs other people. It craves touch, safety, and belonging.

But life has become hectic and your awareness is often occupied with seemingly more pressing matters than the subtle impulse to drink water, lie down, touch someone. You might struggle to notice the cues for thirst, putting off your body's needs for an afternoon. You might try to rationalize away the craving for touch, and instead try to settle for solitude. You might sit at a desk for hours on end without noticing the creak in your back, or the stiffness in your hips.

Your body is talking to you constantly. If you listen, you'll hear the animal communicate its needs. It will tell you if it's in pain. It will tell you when it is comfortable. It will tell you if it's too hot or too cold. It will tell you if something doesn't feel good. It will tell you if it feels unsafe. But, over the last couple of hundred years, modern society has put more and more demands on our bodies, requiring us to be artificially numb to pain, pleasure, and the subtle sensations of being alive. We've become nearly deaf to the voice of the body, ignoring it until it screams so loudly that everything comes to a screeching halt.

To be able to get to your Point B, you have to be able to clearly hear your Body Voice. Life happens in a human body. The work of your life isn't to transcend this body—it's to live *in* it. True transformation happens when—instead of working against your body and treating it like an enemy—you work from within your body, caring for it like you would a sweet animal who needs your attention and care.

## The Language of the Body

The body does not use words or sentences or thoughts. It speaks through physical sensations—often subtle. The body has preferences, opinions, desires, and aversions. Like any other animal, it remembers. It remembers pain, it remembers pleasure. It remembers that falling and skinning your knee felt bad. It remembers that it felt safe in your third-grade teacher's classroom. It remembers that Christmas smells like wood smoke and pine needles and tastes like cinnamon. It remembers the hot plastic waterbed smell in the room where the bad things happened.

It remembers the things you have done to it, the things that were done to it by others, the things that it wasn't allowed, the deprivation it has suffered. It remembers being hungry and not cared for. It remembers being cold, or isolated, or neglected. It remembers being abused through drugs, alcohol, and food. It was there for all of it. When you were in the backseat, checked out and numbed out—Body was there alone for the full brunt of it all.

Your body is not against you. It has patiently, lovingly, been right there with you for your entire life. It communicates to you through tension and relaxation. That sore back? Body is talking. Those stiff legs? Body is talking. That grumbling stomach? Body is talking. That stomachache, headache, coughing fit, sleeplessness, fatigue, exhaustion, restlessness, addiction? Body. Body. Body.

This sounds so simple, right? Eat when you're hungry. Drink when you're thirsty. Rest when you're tired. Navigating the Body Voice sounds straightforward, easy. But—at least for me—this is wildly difficult. Trying to figure out if I'm hungry—like my body actually needs food—or if I just want chips because I'm bored? That's freaking hard. Trying to determine if I should go for a walk or lie down and close my eyes for an afternoon nap? I come up blank. Trying to make myself drink water because I feel thirsty? All I can think is, *Water is boring. Bleh.* Am I getting a cold? Working too hard? Just trying to avoid the hard stuff in life? It's so hard to know.

These nuances can be quite difficult to navigate—so as we move through the Body Voice, we'll keep this as simple as possible. As you dive deeper into your body's subtle wisdom, you'll get clearer on how to use its feedback to guide your way. Eventually, you'll be able to use the voice of your body as a reliable guide.

## On the Mat: Listen to Your Body

To begin with, I'd like you to look at your surroundings through the lens of your animal body. No matter what space you live in, work in, or where you practice yoga—there are places that feel safer, more comfortable, more protected to the animal of your body. You're looking for subtle feedback—maybe even instinctual—what might even feel superstitious, intuitive, or *woo-woo* at first. A dog will lie down in a spot that faces the door. Typically, animals like to feel contained and safe, while being able to see out—so they can assess what might be coming in their direction. Your body is no different. Most human bodies prefer to face looking out through windows rather than having their backs to them. Most human bodies like to be able to maintain their privacy—with the option of pulling the curtains or blinds as it gets dark, rather than feeling like they live in a fish bowl—allowing outsiders to watch them through banks of windows. Where you place your body—and your mat—matters when it comes to accessing the voice of the body. If your body is stressed, or on high alert, it'll be very difficult to hear the subtle information behind the buzz of stress.

Your body knows this intuitively. It knows where it feels safest. Not only for stranger-danger, but also for quick escape in case of fire, flood, or any other environmental threat. It naturally knows if it's trapped or too exposed. It knows if it feels cozy and comfortable or if it feels vulnerable and unprotected.

To begin with, do a quick walk-through of your home and, in general, take an inventory of the safest spaces in your home. Maybe it's the one corner of your couch, or the reading chair near the fireplace. Maybe it's one particular seat at your kitchen table, or your bathtub or your bed. Tune in to your body as you walk through your kitchen, your living spaces, your bathroom. Notice if windows help or hinder the feeling of safety. Notice where the doors are. If you were a deer, or a chipmunk, or a bird, where would you feel safest? Tune in to your inner animal wisdom.

Ask yourself: *What spaces feel best, safest and most comfortable for my body? Why?*

Journal your insights.

Before you even enter my home, you come through a private and pro-tected courtyard. You can't see my home from the street—you have to come through a small gate before you can even see the front door. Without even realizing it, I typically point my body in the direction of that gate when I'm working. Right now, as I type this, I—without even thinking about it—turned my chair to face that gate. The chair is usually positioned fac-ing north, into the conversation pit of my living room. But when I work, I always—unconsciously—face west, toward the entry of my property. My back is to the bedroom where my daughter sleeps—the front of my body is aware and guarding both of us. I don't have to think about doing this—it just feels right. It feels normal. It feels comfortable.

As an experiment—I just tried turning my chair so that my back was to the gate. I felt uncomfortable. It felt like I was in one of those stupid horror flicks where everyone in the audience is shouting, *Look behind you!* My mind knew that there was no Bad Guy lurking out in my garden. But my body became completely occupied with hypervigilance, every hair on my back felt electric. All sensations were on hyperdrive.

To calm my body, all I had to do was turn my chair back around.

Your body—your animal—has preferences. If it's too hot, it might want the safety of having fresh air and an open window nearby. If it's too cold, it might want to be near a fireplace or have a cozy blanket nearby. If it's in a strange place—a hotel room, or new city—it might not feel settled until the general surroundings have been mapped. It might need to know where the stairs are, where the nearest coffee shop is, how it would get out of there in case of emergency before it can settle down. This isn't communicated in sentences, thoughts, or any language that's easy to translate—it might just feel like that creepy back-tingly something's-not-right feeling that I had when I was facing away from the entryway.

Some people call this intuition, some people call this a *gut* feeling (no-tice the body terminology there), some people call this bad feng shui. Whatever you call it, just notice it. Noticing something's *off* is a great start. It's important information—critical to help you be able to connect to your

Four Voices. You can't access the faint sensations of emotion when you are ignoring the needs of the animal. Nor will you be able to settle your mind (let alone your soul) if the animal part of you is panicked.

So, now that you have a general idea of where you feel safest in your house. I'd like you to do a walk-through to figure out what spaces are available for rolling out your mat. Take an inventory of the spaces that might be available for yoga practice and then consider how these spaces feel for the animal of your body.

Roll out your mat in each of these spaces. Take a moment to stand or sit on your mat. Move your arms around and see if you have enough room for your practice. Notice which way you'd want to face, which orientation feels better in the room. Notice if the space feels too tight, too dirty, too cramped, too unsafe, or too exposed.

Ask yourself: *What spaces are available for my practice? What spaces feel the most inviting? Does the area feel comfortable and safe to my body? How do you know the space feels right?*

Journal your insights. You're looking for where you feel safe and comfortable in your home. This is how you acknowledge that you are open to listening to your body's wisdom. I suggest you do this not only with placement of your mat at home but also for where you place your mat in a public class.

Sometimes, as a practice of non-attachment, teachers suggest that people shouldn't stick to their tried-and-true spaces in the yoga studio. Although this might help with non-attachment, this can be very distressing for the body. I have found that the number of people who have abused their body or have had their bodies abused by others are overwhelmingly the majority. If this is you, you need to honor where you feel safest in a room. If that means you always stick to the back left corner, so be it. Please do whatever helps your little animal feel calm and protected.

This also means you stay aware of poses that feel unsafe. You have permission to opt out of any pose that feels risky, unprotected, or just *off* to your body. Even if you have the strength and flexibility to do the pose, you're allowed to protect the animal of your body. Maybe going upside down doesn't feel right to you? Honor that. Maybe balance poses make your heart race and you'd rather stick close to the wall? Honor that, too. You are allowed to take care of your body in any way you see fit, and this doesn't just mean you only watch for physical risks. It means you also respect the intangible risks that might have nothing to do with the pose itself—but might have everything to do with caring for yourself. Notice if something feels off and then do your best to respond in a way that helps your body settle down. When you respond—even just a little—to the voice of your body, you'll notice a visceral trust that unlocks and begins to unfold.

Ask yourself: *What yoga postures have felt unsafe, uncomfortable, or invasive to me? Why?*

Journal your insights.

## Off the Mat: Listen to Your Body

Even if you've been abused, even if you were your own abuser, you still have access to this animal part of you. When you enter an office, a home, a restaurant, a dinner party, or a parking lot, take an inventory of what location feels best within the space. Notice what your body wants—Is your body hot or is it cold? Does it want fresh air or does it want to be contained? Does it want somewhere cozy to sink into or does it want to be able to escape easily?—and respond to those needs.

Ask yourself: *Where do I feel most relaxed, safe, and comfortable? Why?*

No matter where you are, or what situation you find yourself in, you can always check in with the voice of your body and do your best to respond to its needs. The more you practice, the more you'll be able to tap into the deeper layers and the more delicate cues offered by the animal of your body. Journal your findings and notice if you start to see patterns emerge and thank your body for its wisdom.

# chapter nine

# Allowing Body to Guide You

How to use the body's map
while you're awake in the driver's seat.

A friend of mine, after devoting most of her adult life to her career, had found herself at a top position of a large company. Although she'd successfully climbed the corporate ladder, she privately struggled with the company's ethics. She felt protective of her management team yet she'd lost faith in the company. Her mind was fiercely devoted to continuing with her commitment to serve. It argued, "People rely on me! I don't have a choice! I need the income!" Her heart felt intense guilt and fear, it didn't want to let people down, it didn't want to disappoint her managers or tarnish the public's perception of the company.

Her mind stayed steady with its advice. "Carry on with what you're doing," it said. Her heart stayed steady with its advice, "Stay connected and don't let people down." So, she stepped out onstage to deliver the annual corporate report to the shareholders. She lowered the microphone, leaned in to speak, and suddenly burst into a coughing fit. She coughed and choked and paced in circles. She covered her mouth and tried to keep the barking coughs from echoing through the loudspeakers. She tried to drink water, she tried to take breaths, she inhaled sips of air trying to recover. Nothing worked. Every time she started to gain composure, she'd lean toward the microphone and her body broke into coughing spasms again.

Her mind said, *Yes*. Her heart said, *Yes*.

But her body? Body was a big fat: *No!* And when Body says *No*, the body eventually wins.

She never did recover. Eventually someone else took over and she resigned later that day.

To get to your Point B, not only do you need to draw on your mind's wisdom and your heart's sense of direction, but you also need to cooperate with your body. The voice of the body is a quiet force, she's gentle and offers the tiniest of cues while you're trying to navigate. Life takes place within the experience of the animal, so it's crucial you have an open line of communication with the animal of your body.

Remember those kids in the backseat of your little car? Well, Body holds a particularly interesting piece of the puzzle. If she's not happy, if she's not on board with what you're doing, if she's not cared for on your journey—she may go along with you for a little while. She might offer little pieces of information—a stiff neck here, a stomachache there—to start with. But if you continue to ignore her, if you continue to abuse her, if you continue to abandon her, she will pull the emergency brake.

Imagine you adopt a pet—let's make it a puppy so that we're on the same page. This puppy has basic needs; she needs to be fed, she needs water, she needs to feel safe, she needs to know you're there to protect her. Let's just say you're a great caretaker. You provide a safe and secure place for your puppy. You make sure that she is cared for. You stay connected to the puppy and you watch for feedback. You notice when she needs more food. You notice when she needs more water. You notice when she wants to play. You quickly gain a sense of when she needs to pee and poop. You're there for her. You're connected to her.

Now imagine what would happen if you aren't a very good caretaker. Maybe you forget to feed her (or refuse to). Maybe she never really feels safe because you have a hectic schedule and she's not sure when you're going to show up. Maybe you never play with her, or let her go outside. Maybe she's left alone too often and feels isolated and insecure. You're not watching her so you miss the feedback. She grows distant and she stops trusting you. She doesn't know if you're going to be kind to her or if you're going to ignore her. Over time, she stops trying to get your attention. Eventually, depending on how badly she's treated, she might even bite.

It's not hard to guess which animal trusts you more, which animal cooperates with you better, or which animal will be more supportive in getting you to Point B.

Your body has needs—just like a little puppy. And when you don't take care of your body's needs, your journey to any Point B becomes futile.

For many of us, taking care of a pet or a child with attention, love, and care feels easy but we fail to apply the same standards of basic care to our own needs. Most of us have a history of not really caring for (or downright abusing) our bodies. Whether you restricted food, or binged and purged, or overate, or drank too much, or took drugs, or over-exercised, or put your body in unsafe places, or checked out and had meaningless sex, the animal of your body will need patience and kindness so that it can learn to trust you again.

If you suffered neglect or violence or sexual abuse, or if you grew up in a home that never felt all that secure—the animal of your body will need compassion and care so that it can trust you'll prevent this in the future. Whether the abuse or neglect was done by others, or whether it was (unintentionally) done by your own hand, your body needs generosity and attention so that it can recover. You can't expect a dog from the pound to trust you overnight; it has a history you may not know or understand. Likewise, you can't expect your body to just flip a switch and trust you automatically. It'll take time to help your body see you as a caregiver.

## Don't Force

For any animal that's suffered abuse, the first rule is: *Don't force it to do anything it doesn't want to do.* If you have a history of overriding physical sensations and body-based feedback, this can be an incredibly difficult rule to follow. You'll have to drop all of your rules about what your body is supposed to do and about what it's not supposed to do. This includes all your rules about eating, drinking, socializing, resting, playing, and working.

This will require unbelievable amounts of faith—and likewise, your body will need unimaginable amounts of trust.

If you insist on forcing your body to do things it doesn't want to do, you won't be able to listen to the voice of your body. You'll miss her inner guidance and, eventually, the body will stop you in your tracks. Err on the side of kindness. Give up your external rules. Learn the language of your body.

## Keep It Safe

Every animal needs a safe space to rest. It needs a bed or a crate or a cage or a barn or a nest. It needs a place that will keep it sheltered from the elements and protected from predators. Your body needs this, too. It needs a haven—a place where it feels cared for. It needs a place that's a comfortable temperature and protected from the weather—not too hot and not too cold. It needs a comfortable bed, a cozy couch, soft blankets, piles of pillows—whatever helps your body relax and feel nurtured, do what you can to provide this for your body.

This is non-negotiable. There's no way to build a relationship with your body if it doesn't have a place that feels safe and physically comfortable. If you were bringing home a new pet, you'd put care and attention into creating a safe space for her. Offer your body the same kindness.

Your body's voice will offer slight cues—listen for them. If you pay attention, you'll feel a slight relaxation, a coziness, or a comfortable safety. It's going to feel like the difference between wearing something too tight and too short compared to wearing your favorite pair of sweatpants. When you wear something too small or too tight, you might feel uneasy or exposed—but when you wear your comfy sweatpants, you feel loose and comforted.

Touch the blankets, the sheets, the surfaces of things. Notice if they feel good to touch. Notice if your body relaxes or tightens. Stay away from anything itchy, or harsh, or overly sterile. Notice how your body reacts when your surroundings are messy, or if there's too much clutter. It might need protection from chaos and from the demands of modern life. You might notice a softening when you're surrounded by beauty and aesthetically pleasing surroundings. As you get better at listening to the softening of your body, you can fine-tune your surroundings to create the haven your body deserves.

## Give It Water

Beyond providing your pet with a safe environment, you want to make sure that it has access to water and potty breaks. Your body needs the same consideration. So let's keep this as basic as possible. You need to drink water—I'm guessing you already know this. You also need to go to the bathroom. We live in a busy society and many of us trade caring for our body for getting one more thing done on our to-do lists. Listen to your body's needs for water and for bathroom breaks. Your body isn't a machine and its health shouldn't be sacrificed.

Your body tells you when it needs water by signaling a sensation of thirst. It tells you when it needs to pee by signaling an uncomfortable bladder. Start with listening for these basic signals. To mend your relationship with your body, notice when you're thirsty and offer your body water immediately. Notice if you put off taking a bathroom break. Pay attention to what these signals feel like in your body before you attend to them. Take a moment after you drink water or take a bathroom break and notice what your body feels like after you attend to its needs—this is how your body says *thank you* for honoring what it wants. Maybe it feels like a gentle relaxing, or maybe your body feels lighter, or maybe your legs feel less restless— you're looking for tiny cues, little things that might typically go unnoticed. Your body's language says thank you to a bathroom break with the same cues that it will use to say thank you for leaving a toxic job.

## Give It Food

Like any pet, your body needs to be fed. This is a gigantic subject and can be a tricky thing to navigate if you've had a difficult history with food. Libraries of books have been written on the subject of trying to help people navigate the difference between the body's need for food and the emotional or mental attachments to food. I am no expert here and have barely scratched the surface of trying to heal my own relationship with food, so I'll just offer you some simple ideas that have helped me.

First, no animal wants to feel deprived and no animal wants to be forced to do anything. My personal journey with trying to heal my body has come down to promising myself that I will no longer deprive my body. Depriving my body put it into a constant state of stress and fear—it was abusive and I vowed to never treat my body like that again. This was not an easy promise to make, nor was it a simple decision to arrive at. This came out of a lifetime of struggle and really—I'd just come to the end the road. I had tried every diet. I'd tried every restriction. I'd tried every which way of eating and I never found peace. I knew I had to radically change the way I treated my body and I made a pact to no longer scare my body. This meant that I would no longer allow myself to go long stretches without food.

Historically, my body lived in a perpetual state of stress and fear around food—always uncertain as to when I'd stop and care for it. To heal, I made my body a promise—I would feed it, or have food available for it, every few hours. This meant that I had to learn how to grocery shop in a way that would help my animal body settle down. I could no longer just wing it, order out, or pick up take out on my way home. I stocked my fridge and my cupboards with healthy food—a visual symbol that I would not deprive myself. I signed up for vegetable delivery from my nearby farm and put my local farmer's market schedule on my calendar. These were seemingly small changes that made a huge impact on my body's ability to relax. Every time I opened the fridge and saw fresh produce, I could feel my body soften.

Your body will communicate with you about this. For me, this communication was difficult to interpret because I was confused about the sensations that I felt. The sensation that I'd always called hunger turned out to be fear of deprivation. As soon as I was worried about being deprived or being hungry later or being forced to eat certain foods—my body would offer up a distinctly uncomfortable sensation. I'd override this feeling because I'd feel it even if I'd just eaten a meal (because it was fear of deprivation and had nothing to do with the meal I'd just eaten). So, I'd forego eating until the cue for hunger was overwhelming. This led me to a cycle of being over-hungry and then having a difficult time figuring out what, or how much, to eat. My body never felt safe or comforted.

Once I promised myself that I would no longer deprive my body and I got into the habit of stocking my house with healthy foods, something shifted in me. It took a lot of patience, but I no longer felt the fear of deprivation and I found a quieter sensation behind it—an early cue of hunger.

For me, this is where I needed to start. After a childhood of intense physical abuse and a lifetime of food restriction, I started by offering my body little promises for care, for food, for nurturing. I started by trying to listen for the earliest signals of hunger and I responded with feeding my body right away. I did everything I could to help my body trust that I'd no longer deprive it or harm it.

Through these small steps, I started to learn how my body spoke to me. I began to trust my body's wisdom because I could finally rely on it. I could hear it and I could respond to it. This took time and extraordinary amounts of patience but I eventually came to understand how to feed and communicate with the animal I live in.

## Move It

Maybe your body likes to take hikes in the wilderness, or walk through a park. Maybe it prefers to sit on the edge of a beach, or to take a yin class at your local yoga studio. Every animal needs to move, wants to move, enjoys moving. That doesn't mean you have to exert a ton of energy. Rather, this means that your body enjoys being outside of the haven for a little while. If you have a history of rules around exercise, you're going to have to shelve those for a while so you can build trust with your body. (Remember: your body doesn't want to be forced to do anything.)

Your body will communicate when it wants to move. If you pay attention, you might notice an inner restlessness. Often, you'll notice that some part of your body is moving already—you might be tapping your toe, or clicking a ballpoint pen, or fidgeting in your seat. You might also notice your muscles feel tight or contracted, like you need to loosen up. It is a sensation of having energy that wants to move up or out. It might feel like you have an emotional or metaphorical backpack weighing you down, and you just want to take it off. This doesn't mean the cue is dramatic—often it's just a slight sensation of wanting to be outdoors, of wanting to feel the wind on your face, or craving a wider horizon.

If you're not sure, just start off small. You don't need to join a bootcamp, commit to a thirty-day yoga challenge, or train for a marathon. You're wanting, instead, to learn how to read the real-time feedback from your body. Go ahead and go for that walk and if you get tired two minutes into it—no big deal!—just stop. Try a gentle yoga class instead of power yoga. Give yourself permission to drop out of any pose that doesn't feel good. Leave early if your body wants to. Learn the signs of your body—watch how it responds to each pose. Stay connected to it and honor its wisdom.

Your body will talk to you about when it wants to stop. Your legs might feel heavy. You might begin to feel like home is far away. You'll want to slow down or sit down. Your emotional backpack or heaviness might lessen. Your mind might feel more clear. Whatever energy needed to work itself up and out of your body might be gone. You may feel lighter and perhaps even more joyful. This is the body's cue that the movement helped and now it's ready to stop.

The goal here is to learn how to communicate with your body—not to get a specific workout in. Think of this like working with a pet—let your body lead. Let yourself learn what your body wants to do.

## Give It Rest

Every animal sleeps—and you're no different. I used to pride myself on how little sleep I could function on. I used to think that I was doing just fine when I got four or five hours of sleep. It wasn't until I was quite sick that I learned (from my doctor) that I'd need to sleep eight to ten hours a night for about *six months* to try to recover. I thought I was just going to have to go to bed early for one night—I wasn't even close. I had no idea that exhaustion was cumulative in that way. Rest isn't just a quick fix—it's a complete lifestyle change.

"Don't force your animal to do anything it doesn't want to do" takes on an interesting meaning when you look at sleep patterns. For most of my adult life, I'd suffered with bouts of insomnia. I just took this to be *who I was* or *what my body wanted to do*. I thought I was listening to my body when I'd wake up at 2:30, or 3:30 or, if I was lucky, 4:30 and start my day. By noon, I'd need another round of coffee. And often another cup by mid-afternoon.

To heal, though, I had to get radical with this sleep idea. When I found out that I had to stay in bed for all those hours, I panicked. I didn't know how to relax like that. I didn't know how to make my body sleep for that long. Those middle-of-the-night wake-ups were simply a response of being way too stressed for way too long. My body wanted to sleep, but I lived in a way that felt like constant fight-or-flight—making it impossible for my body to feel safe enough to sleep. This had to change.

Sleep is mandatory. It's not a luxury. It's a critical part of taking care of your animal. Start off small. Make yourself a promise that you'll stay in bed for a minimum number of hours. Even if you don't sleep, you'll at least be horizontal. Instead of looking at sleep like something that interrupts the rest of your life, make it a non-negotiable for the animal of your body. Do everything you can to create a safe haven for your body and to communicate to it that it is safe to sleep through the night.

Your body will talk to you about sleep. It already is and you're probably already responding to its cues. If you have a caffeine or sugar habit (especially in the afternoon), notice what makes you go for that cup, or that snack. That impulse is actually the impulse to rest, to sleep—it's feedback from your body that it wants a time-out. Notice when your eyes get heavy at night, when you start to yawn, or when your mind starts to slow down.

Just like any other signal from your body, the more you listen and respond—the easier it becomes. Make sleep a priority and offer your body the opportunity to rest. Notice when or if you reach for sugar or caffeine in the afternoon and see if you can respond with a quick lie down instead.

## Other Things That Help

### Your Body Needs Touch

Humans did not evolve to live alone. They did not evolve to thrive in isolation. Your body knows this. If you live alone, you still need something or someone to love, cuddle, and touch. If that's not an option, commit to regular massages—it's amazing how healing human hands can be for your body. If you live with others, cuddle up, lean on someone, and get a hug.

### Your Body Needs to Feel Protected

No matter how trivial the fear seems to your mind, do what you can to honor your body's fear. Your body starts to shake and shiver when it's afraid. When this happens, listen and do not force it to do anything it's afraid of. Whether it's giving a presentation at work, or going on a first date, notice what's happening to your body. If you notice shaking or shivering or anxiety building—err on the side of kindness. Err on the side of protection. Maybe ask a friend to join you on a double date, or see if someone can take the lead at work. This is about gaining your body's trust—which means to care for it like a child or a pet. If you suffer from any type of social anxiety, or if you notice that your body starts to shake, shiver, sweat, or get nervous around unfamiliar people or in unfamiliar places, protect it from forced interactions. Don't force your body to do anything that it doesn't want to do, and don't try to override your body's fears. Listen to your body, respond to its requests, and be patient.

### Your Body Needs Kindness

Animals—especially dogs and cats—are extremely sensitive to the tone of your voice. Your body is no different. If you're working to heal your relationship with your body, it's best to speak in kind and soft tones to yourself. Do not admonish, do not berate, and do not (even within the privacy of your own mind) verbally abuse your body. This goes for everyone around you. Remove yourself from people who speak harshly about bodies (theirs or yours). Protect the animal and surround your body with support and love.

### Your Body Needs Attention

This is where any relationship starts. It starts with getting to know each other. It starts with building intimacy and trust slowly. It starts with sharing and listening. It starts with kindness and patience. To learn how to listen to your body's wisdom, you'll need to spend some quiet time each day checking in with it. The more you listen to little cues and respond accordingly, the more your body will communicate with you, trust you, and work with you. Make time for some quiet one-on-ones with your body each day to build its confidence and trust in you.

As you get to know your body better, you'll begin to pick up even subtler cues as to what it wants and what it doesn't want. You'll notice that your body relaxes when one person sits down next to you and tenses when a different person sits by you. You'll notice when your body wants a break, wants to go on a walk, wants to work. You'll notice when it's on board with your quest to Point B and you'll notice when it's giving you hints that hinder your progress. You'll be able to listen to this feedback and to respond to it without trying to negate it or override it. Through gentle care, attention, and consistent practice, you'll learn to work with your body as an ally rather than an enemy and you'll be able to tap into the vast wisdom your body holds.

## On the Mat: Shake It Off

*Shake It Off*

When two dogs meet each other, they usually walk around each other, sniff each other's butts—maybe they'll wag their tails or roll over in submission. If they don't like each other, one might raise the fur on her back or the other might bare her teeth. Their muscles will become rigid, ready to fight or protect. They might even bark or nip at the other. When the stress has passed, each dog will continue on her way for a few steps and then she'll do something really interesting.

They shake it off. From head to tail, the entire body wrings itself out to reset and move on. And this isn't just after a conflict, it can happen at any time of the day. If you watch your pets, you might notice that they shake not only after an enemy encounter, but also after they hear a sudden loud noise, or after they bonk into something on accident, or after they wake up from a snooze.

Animals do this instinctually. Once a stress, threat, or surprise has passed, they shake off the muscular tension left over from the encounter. Dogs do this. Cats do this. Hamsters do this. Even hummingbirds do this. The shaking resets their body and restores their nervous system back to a natural, relaxed baseline. No residue is left behind in their muscles. No tension is stored for later.

Your body wants to do this, too. It wants to reset to its relaxed baseline. It wants to relieve itself of tension. It wants to shake it off.

For this practice, you'll need your journal and pen, and some loud music. Dance music and workout playlists are probably too slow for this exercise. This isn't music you're going to bob up and down to, you're looking for something that's wild and faster than you'd typically move to. Take some time to find at least ten minutes of music. Shaking is vigorous and it takes quite a bit of energy—the drum beat will help you keep going.

Before you begin, check in with your body. Move each part of your body so you can feel the joints, the muscles. Check in with how each part of your body feels. Wiggle your fingers and your toes. Start at your feet, and move your awareness through your legs, into your hips. Move your limbs, stretch a little, and check in with the interior of your body. Bring your attention to your digestion, your stomach, and your low back; notice what's happening within. Focus on your core muscles, your back muscles, your shoulders, your neck, your arms, yours hands, and your face. Move, stretch, massage, and palpate to check in with your entire body.

Ask yourself: *Where is my body holding tension? Where is my body tight or stressed?*

Journal your insights.

Find a place in your home where you can move freely. There's no need to stay on a yoga mat for this. Turn the music up and listen to the rhythm.

Begin by shaking your leg. Pick it up and wag it hard. Please know that there's no cool way to do this. You're probably going to look silly. That's okay. You're not shaking to impress your neighbors, friends, or family. This isn't an art form and this isn't choreographed. This is simply a technique of getting the ick off you. Whatever emotional residue you're holding, whatever stress you're hanging onto, whatever pain, stuckness, or exhaustion that's seeped into your body—shake it out.

Shake your foot and your leg. Then shake the other one. Shake your butt and hips like a really fast chicken dance. Shake your shoulders, rib cage, head and neck—think of the *Flashdance* movie in fast motion. Shake your head *yes,* then shake your head *no* as if you're really opinionated at a rapid speed. Let your arms and hands go wild; shake it all out through the tips of your fingers and hands like you're trying to dry yourself off.

Again, you will look like a dork doing this. But trust me, it's so worth it.

Shake and shake and shake. Get it all off of you. Notice any soreness or stiffness and shake it out. Notice where your joints are rickety and shake that out. Don't take yourself seriously; just try to shiver and rattle all the invisible crud away.

Did you have a fight with your sister? Shake it.

Are you stressed about your work deadline? Shake it.

Are you worried about what the neighbors will think when they see you sweating in your jog bra at six in the morning? Shake it.

Do this for a minimum of five minutes.

When you're finished, your heart rate will be elevated, so remain standing until you catch your breath. Scan your body once again. Start with your feet and move to the top of your head. Notice what's changed mentally, emotionally, and physically after shaking. Check in with the pings and creaks you'd found earlier. Move your limbs and joints and observe any changes.

When you're ready, take a seat.

Ask yourself: *What does my body feel like now? How has the quality of my mind, my heart, and my body changed? What are the physical sensations I feel now?*

Journal your insights.

## Off the Mat: Shake It Off

It's helpful to devote part of your yoga practice to include shaking and to treat it as a type of ritual for helping your body reset. You can also take this idea off the mat and incorporate it into your everyday life. Shaking, even just a little bit, helps work emotion out and through so that your body can come back to a neutral and calm baseline.

Try just shaking your hands a few times—like you do when you wash your hands in a public restroom that's out of paper towels. Similar to shaking the water off your hands, shake off anything you want to leave behind. Just two or three quick shakes will do.

This works quickly and can be done completely in the privacy of a car, cubicle, or bathroom stall. If you've had a conflict, fright, or particularly vulnerable experience, you can shake it off. This works for things like getting cut off in traffic—you know those pins and needles that happen in your body after that sudden scare? Shake your hands (one at a time while driving) and help your body reset. If your kids are fighting and screaming and you just can't take one more minute without blowing your fuse, stand right there in front of them and do a full body shake if you're up for it. If not, go hide in your laundry room and shake the frustration away before you enter back into the war zone. If you're freaking out because you have to do a big presentation at work and your pits are sweating through your best suit, find the nearest supply closet or go stand in a bathroom stall and deliberately shake the freak off of your body. If you're feeling anxious—even in the middle of the night—a few vigorous shakes of the hands, while you're still under the covers, might help your body reset so it can sleep.

chapter ten

# The Weird Thing about Pain

How to wake up and chart your course
when Body has taken the wheel.

As a yoga teacher, I'm trained to read bodies. As a coach, I use the body's language to inform me of possible patterns that relate to the realm of the mind, heart, and soul. In large classes where there might be fifty or seventy bodies in the room, I walk row by row while I teach. I look at students' feet in standing poses, the arc of their backs in Child's Pose. I notice muscle tone and flexibility. I notice the person who is straining and forcing a pose. I also notice the person who is checked out and picking at their nails. I notice the people who never allow themselves props, and I notice the ones who flop in and out of their postures—without backbone or purpose. I take mental note of these physical details, just as I do with their personal stories. It's an interesting perspective to take to teach a large class—looking at rows and rows of human animals.

When I'm working with students in my workshops and retreats, their bodies tell me a significant piece of their story. If a student shares that she's having difficulty in her relationship, I'll watch her body language as she speaks. I'll watch her on the mat and off. If I see that she typically walks with tall posture and a strong backbone, her body tells a different story than if she typically holds her head down, collapses her shoulders, and folds her arms in front of her heart.

Without even realizing it, you're reading the stories of the bodies around you, too. When you meet your new cubicle mate and she carries herself in a Wonder Woman stance (think: standing straight, feet slightly apart, broad chest, head high, hands on hips), you will have a different reaction to her than if she appears slumped, in a cowering posture over her desk (think: head down, shoulders rounded, tail tucked, belly loose). One stance naturally feels strong and confident while the other feels insecure and submissive. Before a person even speaks a word, their body has already told you a piece of the story.

## When Body Takes the Wheel

Your own body will tell you a story if you know what to look for and how to listen to it. When you're connected to your body, you'll notice when your body is at ease and you'll notice when it tightens up. When you're listening to the voice of your body, you have access to its instinctual wisdom. It will support you and it will work with you. But as I discussed in the previous chapter, it's easy to forget to listen for these cues, and over time, the line of communication can quickly become compromised.

When you're disconnected or numbed out in the backseat, the three kids—Mind, Heart, and Body—jockey for the wheel. When Mind takes over, your head spins with thoughts trying to control everything to make life predictable and secure. When Heart drives, you live in reaction mode—avoiding pain and chasing pleasure—unconsciously responding to your unrecognized inner emotions. When Body takes the wheel, your life fills with symptoms, ailments, exhaustion, pain, stiffness, and physical unease. Your body doesn't want to drive, she wants to be the container through which you live your life. She wants to work in partnership with you. She gets frightened when she's ignored. So when she's at the wheel, she'll do everything she can to try to get your attention, wake you up, and put you back in the driver's seat.

Body's job is to protect you. First and foremost, that means her job is to keep you alive. When you ignore the body's needs for too long, she will pull the emergency brake and make everything come to a grinding halt. If you go without food, water, or rest, or if you're overworking, she'll handle it for a while. But at some point, the animal will take over and her self-preservation instinct will kick in. If basic needs aren't being met, your body will offer up the usual sensations—thirst, hunger, sleepiness—to get your attention and communicate the need for care. When you don't listen, these cues get louder and more acute.

Your body has needs beyond just being watered and fed. As I shared in the last chapter, your body also has preferences for comfort, safety, touch, and environment. She offers up sensations to try to get your attention about her preferences. If your body doesn't like your job, your boss, doesn't feel safe in your home, or hates air conditioning, she will talk to you about this, offering physical sensation as feedback. And when you jump into the backseat, numb out, or override these cues, she resorts to other techniques to get your attention. In extreme cases, where you've ignored your body for way too long, she'll stop the journey through extreme fatigue, sickness (brief or chronic), or debilitating pain such as a back going out or a migraine. This isn't because she's angry and it isn't because she's trying to punish you. Her job is to protect you. When she stops you in your tracks, she's trying to save your life.

## Your Body Tells a Story

If your body doesn't want to park in the underground garage, you'll feel a nervousness or a shiver. If she doesn't want to sit long hours in front of a computer, you'll feel stiffness and soreness in your spine. If she doesn't want to run five miles today, you'll feel tired and heavy. When you're connected to this voice and listening closely, you'll notice that you feel particularly drained after a certain meeting, or you'll notice that your body sweats and shakes when you board an airplane. You'll feel a sense of physical attraction or relaxation with a person and a sense of disgust or unease with someone else.

When you're not listening, your body offers louder messages. I'm not saying that if you get a sliver in your pinky finger, your body is communicating some deep-seated truth. Sometimes, a sliver is a sliver, a stubbed toe is just a stubbed toe, and coming down with a cold is just the luck of the draw. But sometimes, these things aren't just random occurrences. Sometimes, your body is communicating an important message.

Whether you're in a boardroom, a doctor's office, or sitting in the lobby of a bank, sometimes you just feel something weird in the air. Maybe someone is fighting, hiding something, or is deeply upset—you pick up on these cues. There's an icky residue in the space whether the person is there or not.

Animals sense danger. Even if your pet has never been to a vet, you'll see them start to get nervous as they get closer to the door. There's something in the air—a smell, a pheromone, a residue—that puts them on high alert. Your body is no different. It sorts through countless pieces of unseen information every second of every day and alerts you to possible dangers and threats. Your body also senses safety and calm. If you create a conscious awareness of when you feel at ease, when you feel your shoulders settle and your breathing relax, you will begin to sense the relationships that you trust, the places where you feel most at home.

A friend of mine is the quintessential definition of conflict-avoidant. When she found herself involved in an explosive lawsuit, she did everything she could to try to bypass, dodge, and escape the inevitable. She didn't want to fight. She didn't want the strife. She wanted to believe that she could solve her problems peacefully and passively. Regardless of her best efforts to come to an amicable solution, the lawsuit wouldn't go away. Within a few months, it festered into an aggressive personal attack that threatened her personal assets as well as her business.

The more hostile it became, the more she retreated into denial. She tried to busy herself at work. At night, she numbed out with wine, binge-watching season after season of *Breaking Bad*. This worked in the evenings, but the following morning she would wake to face the ever-burgeoning piles of paperwork and the imminent conflict looming on the horizon.

A few months into this, she woke up and one of her eyes was swollen shut. It was painful and crusty and she couldn't open it. She had no idea what had happened to her eye—she wasn't sick, it hadn't been hurt, the pain had come out of nowhere. Each day her eye got worse, the pain made it impossible for her to see. She tried hot compresses, cold washcloths, massaging her brow, and a variety of eyedrops. No matter what she did, her eye continued to fester and sting. After a few days of this, her other eye became swollen and irritated. The following morning, she woke to both eyes swollen shut. She went to the doctor and was told that she'd just been really unlucky—that these things happen sometimes. She was told to rest and wait it out.

I offered the suggestion that her body might be trying to communicate with her. I'd watched her avoid her lawsuit for months and had witnessed the toll it had taken on her emotionally and physically. I asked her if she saw a connection: "Do you think this might be related to the lawsuit? Do you think your body might symbolically be showing you how painful it is to keep your metaphorical eyes shut?"

She sheepishly confessed that this was probably true. Admitting this seemed to click a switch in her. She knew she could no longer avoid the truth—she had to engage in the conflict. She had to protect her assets. She had to fight. She heard her body's message and resolved to move forward. That day, she made a series of phone calls, and got a court date scheduled. Her body responded immediately. Within twenty-four hours, the swelling began to subside. Her eyes, still painful, were finally able to open a little. She stopped numbing out at night, threw away the wine, and began studying her court case in the evenings. She made notes and came up with a strategy. Within days, her eye had completely cleared. No swelling. No pain. Eyes wide open.

Her body had a message: it didn't want to ignore the problems any longer. It knew the burden that she was bearing. Even though she was doing her best to ignore her lawsuit, to numb her fear and to avoid the conflict, the animal of her body never left her side. Her body felt the emotion that she ignored and it endured the stress and tension that she'd failed to address. When she jumped in the backseat with her wine and Walter White, her body never abandoned her and did its best to get her attention. Her body wasn't on board with her habit of denial and offered up a physical message to show her how detrimental her conflict-avoidance had become.

I've had many students who have a difficult time setting boundaries, but one, Lisa, stood out as an ultimate people-pleaser. She almost never said no. She volunteered for her church every weekend. She was an active member of her daughter's PTA. She worked full time at a demanding corporate job. She stayed up late helping her husband work on his book and woke up early to take care of the family pets. Between church and kids and husband and pets and work, she had no personal time. She lived in reaction mode; if anyone asked her to do anything, she'd automatically say yes.

She had a difficult and painful relationship with her mother. There were no borders to where her mother's life ended and where Lisa's life began. If her mother needed her, Lisa would drop everything and get on a plane to be by her side. No matter how great the sacrifice, her mother never seemed to be pleased with her. Lisa craved her mother's love and affection, but the only attention she received was through demands and criticisms. Her mother would comment about Lisa's weight, her hair, what she wore, who she married, what she did for a living—there was no end to the laundry list of shortcomings.

Lisa never said a word. She'd just listen and nod and do her best to forgive and forget. She'd come back from the visits browbeaten and shame-ridden—but eventually, she'd slap on a smile and get back to her busy routine.

As we worked together, Lisa began claiming her life back. She began saying no to things she didn't love. She began carving out time for herself. Little by little, she learned to use her voice and speak up for what she wanted.

A few months later, Lisa's mother called from the airport, luggage in hand, announcing her arrival for a surprise visit. Lisa hadn't planned for this, nor was she prepared for this. She couldn't bring herself to admit the truth of how she felt—even within her own mind. She didn't want her mom there, but she would never disclose her secret feelings. She felt guilty and responsible and like she had no choice. She drove to the airport and brought her mom back home with her.

Her mother started in on the car ride home, commenting on her hair color—*well, it covers the gray but the red makes your skin look pasty*, her husband's weight—*does he still have that Santa belly*, her kids' grades—*they'll never get into the Ivy League with those grades*. Her mother picked and pecked her way through the entire first evening. Lisa said nothing. She just quietly seethed. Boiling in resentment, she did her best to bury her feelings. She tried to forgive and forget. She went to bed early and hoped that the following day would be better.

The next morning she woke up and found she had no voice. She didn't have a sore throat, and she didn't seem to have a cold, but she had a case of laryngitis that rendered her speechless. She was only able to speak in soft whispers and even that was difficult. She sent me an email asking, "Do you think the laryngitis has anything to do with my boundary issues with my mom?"

Lisa intuitively knew that her body had a message for her. She couldn't speak. Being rendered voiceless had made her mother's visit intolerable. She was mute, but the onslaught of insults kept coming. She wanted to scream, but couldn't.

I wrote back, "Ask your body."

Lisa shared later that her body had given her a clear message: not speaking is painful, intolerable, debilitating. The laryngitis had given her tangible proof of how much she needed to use her voice. Lisa ended up grabbing a Sharpie to write across a Post-It note, "Mom, you need to go home," and carried the note out to her mother. Her mother pushed back with her typical shame-and-guilt tactics. But Lisa steadfastly held the Post-It note in response. She didn't waiver. Eventually, her mother huffed, packed up her luggage, and went home.

As you can probably guess, Lisa's voice came back the following day.

## What Is Your Body Trying to Say?

Does this mean that Lisa's laryngitis, or my friend's swollen eyes, were all in their heads? Does this mean that they brought these ailments on themselves as some kind of self-sabotage? Does this mean you can heal anything by just talking to your body? No, no, and no. The symptoms, pain, styes, laryngitis—these are real things that happen. The pain is real. The suffering is real. The symptoms and ailments are real. Yours are, too.

That said, there are times when symptoms appear to relate to personal, emotional, and psychological challenges. I invite you to consider both the causal and the symbolic when your body offers pain, ailments, or symptoms. First, start with getting medical advice from a trusted health care provider. Then, consider the possibility of a metaphorical or symbolic message from the Body Voice.

For example, if you tear your Achilles tendon, by all means get yourself to a doctor. And after you do, look into the myth of Achilles. The myth may remind you that you might be emotionally, financially, physically, or spiritually at risk. It might be a warning to protect your weak spot—your metaphorical Achilles' heel—and that you must try to protect what's most vulnerable to you.

You're not looking for a quick fix, but rather looking to initiate a conversation with your body. There's no right way to do this, and there are no right answers to find. Your body isn't trying to punish, hurt, hinder, or chastise you. It's merely trying to protect you.

Ask your body: *What are you trying to tell me? What message are you trying to convey?*

And then wait. Your body's messages might be difficult to understand. It might take hours, days, or years to really understand your body's message.

Years ago, I suffered through months and months of debilitating vertigo. Every time I moved my head, I'd get dizzy and lose my balance. It felt like the ground was falling out from under me. I couldn't do yoga and I could only drive if I kept my head perfectly still. I'd wake up in the middle of the night, feeling like I was falling—only to discover that I was safe in bed. I went to my healthcare provider and there was nothing she could do. We tried medication and we tried vertigo head maneuvers—but nothing worked.

Day in and day out, I asked my body, *What are you trying to tell me? What message are you trying to convey?* I'd write in my journal, "The only message I keep finding is that things are unstable, the ground isn't real." This made no sense. At the time, life seemed good. I was dating a guy I really liked. He seemed stable and honest and I was optimistic about our future together. After a few months, the vertigo went away, just as quickly as it came on. But then a few months later, it came back again with a vengeance.

I asked my body again and got the same responses: things are unstable, the ground isn't real. This feedback still didn't make any sense to me and I didn't end up having any epiphany that miraculously healed my vertigo. For the next year, I had vertigo that came and went every few months.

However, months after I finally ended that relationship, I found out that he had been keeping some very significant secrets. Secrets that had put me and my daughter in danger. Secrets that had, unbeknownst to me, made our lives very unsafe. His secrets had started around the time my vertigo set in. At the time, I had no conscious idea of what he'd been up to, but it seems that my body did know something and had tried to get my attention. The metaphorical ground I had been standing on was unstable and wasn't real.

I've seen too many bizarre body stories to discount the profound ways that our bodies communicate. So I teach my students to take a half-and-half approach to listening to their body. Anytime you find a ping, pain, ache, or ailment, first consider that your body is experiencing something purely medical, coincidental, and circumstantial. Always follow up on real concerns about pain or illness with a medical provider first. Then, reflect on the possibility that your body is simply offering up a symbolic, metaphorical message to get your attention related to something psychological or emotional. By reaching out to your doctor and simultaneously opening up a dialogue with yourself, you are paying attention to the truth of what is going on for your body and reaching for the most healthy outcome.

If you have a hunch your pain might be your Body Voice talking but you're stuck and can't decipher the message, here are some of the things I've found helpful:

### It Might Be Trauma

In *The Body Keeps the Score*, where the very title of the book points to the direct relationship between your body and your history, Bessel Van Der Kolk states, "Physical self-awareness is the first step in releasing the tyranny of the past."[10] If you have trauma or abuse in your past, this book is a must. Dr. Van Der Kolk shows how trauma changes the brain and the body. Those who have experienced profound trauma need more than talk therapy; they may need to learn or relearn—in a safe and gentle way—how to feel the sensations in their body. Dr. Van Der Kolk says, "The act of telling the story doesn't necessarily alter the automatic physical and hormonal responses of bodies that remain hypervigilant, prepared to be assaulted or violated at any time. For real change to take place, the body needs to learn that the danger has passed and to live in the reality of the present."[11] You may have already gone to a therapist for your old stuff. But if you didn't work with someone who helped you connect back to your body, you might need to try someone, such as a somatic therapist, who specializes in helping you build a bridge to your body.

### It Might Be Camouflage

Your pain might be concealing unconscious issues. Beyond keeping you physically alive, your body often has a very interesting and mysterious job of protecting you from emotional and psychological pain. The Body Voice acts kind of like the oldest sister to the three kids in the backseat. If things get too tough for Heart or Mind, Body takes over for them. She offers up a smoke screen of physical sensation to keep the deeper pain hidden. The idea that pain means injury or damage is deeply ingrained in our consciousness. Of course, if your leg starts hurting while you're running, it's natural to think that the pain was caused by running. But as I mentioned before, this isn't always the case.

In *Healing Back Pain*, Dr. John E. Sarno says that the role of pain is "not to express the hidden emotions but to prevent them from becoming con-

---

10. Van der Kolk, *The Body Keeps the Score*, 101.

11. Ibid., 21.

scious." He goes on to say that sometimes pain is created "to distract the attention of the sufferer from what is going on in the emotional sphere. It is intended to focus one's attention on the body instead of the mind." [12]

According to Dr. Sarno, sometimes pain (and when I say pain I mean any type of pain including chronic pain, autoimmune syndromes, irritable bowel syndrome, allergies, headaches and migraines, eczema, psoriasis, acne, hives, and much more) is actually serving as a camouflage to deeper things hidden in our subconscious. Basically, it works like this: Something really scary or awful happened and your body goes to work throwing up a big smoke screen or distraction (called pain) to, in effect, cover your eyes so you don't have to deal with that scary or awful thing.

In cases like this, the role of the pain isn't to express the hidden emotions but to prevent them from becoming conscious. It's created to distract you from what is going on in the emotional sphere, so that you're focusing all of your attention on the physical pain instead of the emotional pain hidden beneath it. It's a fancy diversion tactic. By the way, virtually no one suffering from this kind of sensation thinks, in the moment, that their pain is related to emotional factors. Almost everyone thinks it's related to injury, congenital or degenerative abnormalities, or external irritants (like in the case of allergies). As long as your focus remains on the pain, there is no danger that the emotions will be revealed. And get this! The really weird thing is that when you're taught what's really going on, when you learn how to call pain's bluff, the pain and its symptoms often disappear.

### Turn to Ancient Wisdom

If I drew a map of a body and asked you to point to the location of heartbreak, I'm guessing you wouldn't point to the earlobe; instead, you'd probably point to the middle of the chest. You experience heartbreak in the exact same physical location I do—in the same place all humans do—right around your heart. We use phrases such as *it's in my blood, down to my bones, heavy heart, punch to the gut,* and *blindsided* for a reason: our language organically points us back to patterns of physical experience within

12. John E. Sarno, *Healing Back Pain: The Mind-Body Connection* (New York: Grand Central Publishing, 1991), 56.

our body. These aren't just metaphorical or coincidental, these phrases help us to name our collective experience.

Your body organizes feelings and stores memories into reliable (and predictable) areas of the body. This wisdom (called the chakra system) originated in India between 1500 and 500 BC in the ancient texts called the Vedas, and continues to be used to this day in meditation, yoga, and ayurveda (one of the world's oldest holistic healing systems). Like feelings or thoughts, chakras can't be held like a physical object, yet they have a strong effect upon the body. If you have tight hamstrings, low back pain, or a stomachache, these are clues pointing the way to hidden messages within the body. Your body predictably holds things such as fear, shame, anger, and sadness in specific places. If you have tightness, congestion, or illness in these hubs, your body might be holding onto stuck emotions, stories, or thought patterns.

## On the Mat: Give Your Body What It Needs

I suggest having your favorite props nearby—you might use bolsters, blankets, blocks, straps, or towels. You'll also need your journal and a pen. This practice focuses on four different centers in your body—legs, hips, core, and chest. As you move through these poses, notice which postures feel easy, uninhibited, or comfortable and which feel congested, difficult, or uncomfortable.

*Wide-Legged Forward Fold—Prasarita Padottanasana*
Come to a Wide-Legged Forward Fold. Hold on to opposite elbows so that your upper body can hang and relax like a rag doll. This should feel easy and stable rather than full of effort. For a greater range of motion, bend your knees slightly. Slow and deepen your breath. Find stillness as you relax deeper into the pose. Hold the pose for about three minutes.

While in the pose, scan your body and notice any sensations you feel in your feet, the backs of your legs, your neck, and across your back. Notice what your head feels like to hang there. Close your eyes and move your focus into the interior of your physical body. Notice the pace of your breath, your heart rate. As you spend more time in this pose, bring your attention to the voice of your body. Rather than focusing on your thinking mind, or emotional state, check in specifically with the sensations you feel in your body.

Ask yourself: *Does my body like this? What would make this feel better for my body?*

You might find that your body loves this pose, but it might feel better for you to use a prop, bend your knees even more, or come out of the pose a little. Work with your body and respond to its feedback. Notice what happens within the pose when you listen to your body's feedback and respond. Notice if your muscles tense or relax, notice if you become more or less flexible.

Journal your insights.

### Cobbler's Pose—Baddha Konasana

Next, check in with your hips in Cobbler's Pose. If your hips are tight, raise your seat by folding a blanket or towel under you. Bend your knees and bring the soles of your feet together. Notice the sensation in your outer hips and relax your legs so that your knees move to or toward the floor. Don't force your legs to open; rather, relax and allow them to unfold to a place with a comfortable amount of sensation. If you want to go deeper, bend forward from your hips, extend your spine, and bring your torso toward your feet without rounding your back. Bring your attention to the sensation in your hips. Hold the pose for about three minutes.

While in the pose, scan your body and notice any sensations you feel in your legs, your neck, and across your back. Close your eyes and move your focus into the interior of your physical body. Notice the pace of your breath, your heart rate.

Ask yourself: *Does my body like this? What would make this feel better for my body?*

If you find that this pose is a bit uncomfortable, check in with your body to determine if there's anything that might help create more space in this pose. Try lifting your seat by sitting on a towel or a blanket. Notice how your body responds. You might also try rolling up towels and placing support under your knees, allowing your legs to relax. Work with your body and respond to its feedback. Notice if your muscles tense or relax. Notice the difference between how your body responded to this pose compared to the previous pose.

Journal your insights.

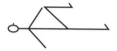

### Twist—Supta Jaṭhara Parivartānāsana

Lie down on your back with your knees bent and your feet flat on the floor. Draw your right knee toward your chest. Place your left hand on the outside of your right knee. Take a big inhale. As you exhale, drop your right knee over the left side of your body into a gentle twist. Do not force your body. Simply notice the sensation as you twist deeper into the stretch. Allow yourself to relax into the floor. Hold the pose for about three minutes.

While in the pose, scan your body and notice any sensations you feel in your legs, your torso, your hips, your neck, and across your back. Close your eyes and move your focus into the interior of your physical body.

Ask yourself: *Does my body like this? What would make this feel better for my body?*

Even if you feel completely comfortable in this pose, challenge yourself to see if your body offers any feedback that would make this pose even better. Maybe it wants a pillow, maybe it wants more support. Maybe your feet are cold and your body wants you to put socks on. As your scan your body, listen to its cues and respond to its feedback. Notice what happens within the pose when you listen to your body's feedback and respond.

Journal your insights. And repeat the twist and inquiry on your left side.

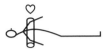

*Restorative Heart Opener*

Start with a rolled blanket or towel as your prop. As you move deeper into this pose and listen to your body's feedback, you might find you want to increase the intensity by using a bolster or block. To begin with, place a rolled towel across your back, perpendicular to your spine, at the bottom of your shoulder blades, right around your bra strap. Lie down on your back, allowing yourself to relax over the prop into a gentle, restorative chest-opening backbend. Your legs can be in any position—outstretched, knees bent with feet flat on the floor, or knees bent with the soles of your feet together. Stretch your arms overhead, elbows slightly bent, and allow them to relax on the floor. Hold the pose for about three minutes.

While in the pose, scan your body and notice any sensations you feel in your legs, your torso, your chest, your shoulders, your neck, and across your back. Close your eyes and move your focus into the interior of your physical body.

Ask yourself: *Does my body like this? What would make this feel better for my body?*

If you want to deepen the chest opening, replace your blanket with a bolster or a block. Check in with your body and notice what happens as you increase or decrease the back bend. Listen for feedback from your body. Maybe you notice your legs become tighter, or your breathing becomes more shallow—if so, respond to your body's feedback and lessen the intensity of the pose. Notice what happens within the pose when you listen to your body's feedback and respond. Notice if your muscles tense or relax, notice if you become more or less flexible. Notice the difference between how your body responded to this pose compared to the previous poses.

Journal your insights.

## Off the Mat: Give Your Body What It Needs

Off the mat, you can use this inquiry in any situation to help forge a stronger connection with the voice of your body.

Ask yourself: *Does my body like this? What would make this feel better for my body?*

Check in with yourself at work. You might find that your body doesn't like the placement of your desk, or that it wants a better chair, or that it would rather work outside. Maybe your body wants different lighting, more windows, a different temperature, or hates your commute. By checking in with your body and responding to its feedback, you'll strengthen your connection to your Body Voice, allowing you to feel more relaxed, capable, and clear while you're working.

Check in with yourself about what you eat. Ask yourself: *Does my body like this?*

This isn't about how something tastes—we all know that candy and chips taste great—it's about how your body responds to them. If you feel bloated, gassy, lethargic, constipated, or nauseous after eating, your body doesn't like it. Even if it's a food that's supposedly good for you, pay attention to how your body feels after you eat something. There are all kinds of "healthy" foods (for example, broccoli, cauliflower, lentils, and legumes) that might be really uncomfortable for your body to digest. Do what you can to connect to your body's experience of a particular food and listen to its feedback and wisdom. There are also a lot of foods that might taste great but might make your body feel bad later. To care for your animal, you want to listen to its feedback and help to protect it from feeling bad.

Ask yourself: *What would make this feel better for my body?*

This might mean you eliminate a particular food from your diet, or that you cut way back. It might also mean you add in more of something that it loves.

Check in with yourself about a situation. For any situation, it can be extremely helpful to simply check in with your body. Your body holds tremendous wisdom and will communicate with you about its preferences. You can use this inquiry for small things such as, *Do I want to go to yoga tonight?* Or for big things such as, *Do I want to get married?* This doesn't mean you base your life choices solely on your body's feedback. But rather, that you take your body's needs into consideration as you move forward through your decision-making process. As you practice wayfinding by listening to your body's cues, you'll notice the sensations of tightness and resistance that happen when your body doesn't like something. When you're working in harmony with your body, you'll feel your body let go and relax, and you'll begin to experience lightness and ease within.

# Wayfinding with Your Body Voice

Through inquiry, you'll first take an inventory of your body's current needs. Without scanning your body to assess its basic needs and attending to those first, you won't be able to move into the subtler feedback your body offers about a specific situation. The wayfinding practice is to stay present while you experience the physical sensations present in your body, to become aware of what your body might need in the present moment, and to learn to trust that you can work together with your body as you journey to Point B. Although certain sensations might be more dominant, your body may have a long list of concerns. In every situation, you should bring your attention to the full spectrum of physical sensations your body presents. Even if you're not consciously aware of these sensations, through inquiry you may find that they are indeed present in your Body Voice—offering even deeper wisdom than what might be noticeable on the surface.

## Body Inquiry Method

### Set an intention to have a conversation with your body.

If you were meeting a close friend for coffee to hear her exciting or terrible news, you would pull up a chair, be quiet, and deeply listen. Imagine that you can just sit down and have this same close conversation with your body—the idea is to simply open up a dialogue. By setting an intention, you focus your attention on receiving your body's wisdom. Do not overthink things, there is no right or wrong way to do this. Do your best to stay aware of your physical body throughout this inquiry practice. Be gentle and patient with your body—take it slow and observe the subtle. Simply state to yourself—out loud or in your head—*I intend to have a conversation with my body.*

### Take a full inventory of your body as it is in the present moment.

Take a few deep breaths. Check in with your feet, legs, hips, back, core, chest, shoulders, arms, hands, neck, and head. Check in with your skin, digestion, breathing, and heart rate. Is your body thirsty? Hungry? Tired? Hot or cold? Is it uncomfortable for any reason? Do your clothes feel comfortable? Do you need a bathroom break? Are all of your body's needs addressed at the current moment? Record anything you find.

### Respond to your body's basic needs.

If you're thirsty, get some water. If you're hungry, eat something nourishing. If you're tired, find a comfortable place to rest. To be able to listen for the subtle feedback of your Body Voice, you must first come to a comfortable place where your body's needs have been cared for.

### Look for symbolic or metaphorical messages.

Take a full inventory of any ailments, illnesses, injuries, pains, or symptoms. If you have underlying symptoms, ask your body if there are any symbolic or metaphorical messages it's trying to communicate. Record any images, insights, or ideas that come to you. You may not have any immediate answers that come to mind. That's okay. The primary purpose of this inquiry process is to set the intention of opening a dialogue with the Body Voice. Physical symptoms may or may not give you feedback on the particular situation in question, but it is still important to note how your body feels. The more you become attuned to all of the sensations and messages of your physical body, the better you will become at checking in with the Body Voice on a regular basis.

### *What's the situation?*

Now that you've checked in with your body and addressed any present needs, you can move on to checking in with your body for navigation. Whether you're wanting to clarify a difficult situation, get to your version of Point B, make a decision, or find your way when you're entirely lost, start with articulating your situation. In just a sentence or two, write a short version of your dilemma, quandary, or story.

### *Regarding this situation, what does your body want?*

Sometimes, the answer will sound like a sentence in your head—like what you'd expect from your Mind Voice. That's okay, just go with it. Sometimes the answer comes through as a physical sensation. A sense of tightening, a tensing, or a feeling of resistance in your body most often means that your body doesn't agree with what you're asking. A sense of relaxation, comfort, or a feeling of ease in your body most often means your body does agree with what you're asking. If you're stuck and aren't able to decipher your body's feedback, keep returning to your breath work. Connection with the body—especially if we are out of practice—can require patience. If no clear message comes to you, you might consider how your body has historically responded to similar situations. In hindsight, what did your body want then?

### *What would make this situation feel easier, more comfortable, kinder, or safer for your body?*

Your body is an animal and wants to work with you. It is a willing companion when it can depend on you to offer kindness, compassion, and safety. Consider your body's physical needs for food, water, rest, movement, sleep, and touch. Reflect on your body's current level of health, what special considerations it might need at this point in time.

### *Specify your Point B for this particular situation.*

Think about the big picture here and articulate your larger intention, focus, commitment, and priority.

### *Is Body's advice taking you to where you want to go?*

Reflect on how your body responds to the situation. Notice if it resists the situation, or if it feels tired or exhausted by the situation. Your body will have preferences. Sometimes these preferences seem to contradict your overall plan to get to Point B. This might mean your body knows something that is still unconscious to you. Or, it might mean you'll have to give a little more consideration for how you care for your body as you move toward your Point B.

### *What can you do to honor your body's wisdom as you journey to Point B?*

Maybe you offer your body more rest, more time off, better food, or more time outside. Maybe you make some hard choices with your boundaries—protecting your body from toxic relationships, toxic work environments, or unhealthy lifestyle choices. Brainstorm ideas and then check in with your body; notice when it relaxes or offers a sense of ease or flexibility.

### *Thank Body and move her to the backseat.*

Here's your new script: "Thank you, Body, for trying to keep me healthy and safe. I will do my best to honor your input. My larger intention, focus, commitment, and priority is _____. I will stay connected to your wisdom as I move in that direction."

## Quick Review of the Body Inquiry Method

1. Set an intention to have a conversation with your body.
2. Take a full inventory of your body as it is in the present moment.
3. Respond to your body's basic needs.
4. Look for symbolic or metaphorical messages.
5. What's the situation?
6. Regarding this situation, what does your body want?
7. What would make this situation feel easier, more comfortable, kinder, or safer for your body?
8. Specify your Point B for this particular situation.

9. Is Body's advice taking you to where you want to go?

10. What can you do to honor your body's wisdom as you journey to Point B?

11. Thank Body and move her to the backseat. Here's your new script: "Thank you, Body, for trying to keep me healthy and safe. I will do my best to honor your input. My larger intention, focus, commitment, and priority is _____. I will stay connected to your wisdom as I move in that direction."

### Example: Emotional Overwhelm

1. **Set an intention to have a conversation with your body.**

2. **Take a full inventory of your body as it is in the present moment.** I was hungry and thirsty—so first I drank some water and ate lunch. My body still feels really tired and wants to just sleep.

3. **Respond to your body's basic needs.** My body seems to be screaming for rest and comfort. So I put on my pajamas, pulled the curtains shut, and jumped into bed. Immediately, I can feel my body relax and a flood of exhaustion move through my body. The darkness feels so much better than bright sunlight.

4. **Look for symbolic or metaphorical messages.** My eyes are killing me. They are stinging and are sensitive to the light. The only thing that feels better is to pull the curtains and close my eyes. Metaphorical message seems to be: close your eyes.

5. **What's the situation?** I'm feeling torn and overwhelmed. I have so many things to do but I'm also exhausted and just want to sleep.

6. **Regarding this situation, what does your body want?** My body definitely wants to rest. But my mind is busy listing all the things that need to be done. I have dozens of emails I need to respond to and hours of work still out in front of me. But Body is clear—it wants to rest.

7. **What would make this situation feel easier, more comfortable, kinder, or safer for your body?** There are a couple of high-priority

things that need to be done today. I can work in my pajamas, in bed, in the dark room to help address my body's needs.

8. **Specify your Point B for this particular situation.** To live a healthy life.

9. **Is Body's advice taking you to where you want to go?** Yes. If I trust my body, I think closing my eyes and resting will help me live a healthier life.

10. **What can you do to honor your body's wisdom as you journey to Point B?** When I feel this type of exhaustion, I can honor my body by going to bed, drawing the curtains and taking the rest of the day off. Instead of pushing through, or setting unhealthy expectations for work, I can just stop and rest immediately.

11. **Thank Body and move her to the backseat.** "Thank you, Body, for trying to keep me healthy and safe. I will do my best to honor your input. My larger intention, focus, commitment, and priority is to live a healthy life. I will stay connected to your wisdom as I move in that direction."

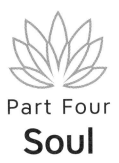

## Part Four
# Soul

The Soul Voice is the intangible essence of your being. This voice knows who you are beyond your ego, your programmed beliefs, your mind, your emotions, and even your body. This is the voice that is not only connected to the deepest and truest sense of who you really are but is also simultaneously connected to who you've always been and who you will become. The voice of the soul often sounds like a compassionate adult speaking to a small child.

As we move through the next few chapters, you'll learn tools to help you listen to the voice of your soul. I'll show you how to find your way using Soul's compass, and I'll show you how to move forward when your inner light goes dark.

# chapter eleven

# The Soul Voice

An introduction to the voice of the soul.
How it works, how to recognize it,
and how it influences your journey.

On your way to Point B, the three kids in the back—Mind, Heart, and Body —share pieces of the map. Mind holds a map that helps you rationally determine where to go. Heart holds a map that guides you through emotional direction. And Body holds a map that helps you stay alive and safe on your journey. If you are present and stay in the driver's seat, you have access to their guidance. If you disconnect and jump in the backseat, the three kids take turns steering your life.

Soul works in a different way. She doesn't hold a map, and she's not duking it out with the kids in the backseat. Instead, she sits quietly in the passenger seat with her compass. Her compass doesn't point north nor does it direct you to Point B. Soul's compass points in a direction that often feels nonsensical, mysterious, or downright confusing. Her compass sometimes points in the exact opposite direction that every other part of you wants to go.

So where does the soul's compass point? Well, that depends.

Sometimes it points to a place that I call *warmer*. Do you remember that game when we were kids called Warmer-Colder? That game where you're trying to get somewhere (maybe you're blindfolded) and the other person says *warmer* when you're getting closer, and *colder* when you move away?

Well, sometimes Soul's compass works something like that. Other times, the soul's compass seems to be entirely random and nonsensical. At times like those, it's almost as if the soul is holding less of a compass and more of a Magic 8-Ball—yes, the black plastic toy you may or may not have used as your own personal fortune teller once upon a slumber party. And then there are times where the soul's compass points in a direction that completely turns your life upside down. I call this direction the Toto Effect—as in Dorothy's Toto—because it's the direction that drives the story (aka your life) forward.

In the next chapter, we'll dive deeper into the details of this compass, how it works, how to use the Soul Voice for guidance, and whether or not that guidance will get you to Point B. For now, I just want you to know that Soul's sitting shotgun and sorta-kinda offers guidance ... sorta-kinda sometimes. Frustrated yet? Yep, me too. But, the good news is you can hone your Soul Voice listening skills—and through practice, you'll be able to access the Soul Voice as readily as any other of the Four Voices.

## What Is the Soul?

Soul isn't your guardian angel nor does she sound like Morgan Freeman (although, wouldn't *that* be cool?). Rather, I think of the Soul Voice as a voice that comes from the part of you who has access to a bigger perspective. Call it the Real You, the More Divine You, the Enlightened You, or the Whole-Healed-Wide-Awake You. It's the voice that comes from the part of you that's not bound by the confines of time, space, or rationality. It's the voice that seems to be able to connect to a greater, universal, or divine intelligence.

Before we go on, let me put you at ease. The Soul Voice can definitely be interpreted as a God type of voice. I don't teach it that way, because it seems a little reckless to give any one of the Four Voices that much power. You have your own unique relationship to this voice. For you, this voice might relate to God—or it might not. I leave it to you to determine what feels true. After teaching this voice for many years, I've found that most students do not see the Soul Voice in a way that relates to a particular religion, spiritual practice, or certain philosophy. Rather, they come to see the Soul Voice as the voice with a bird's-eye point of view, the voice that connects you to something larger than your current situation.

## The Inner Flame

When I talk about the Soul Voice, I'm talking about the information that comes from your highest inner consciousness. In some traditions, this part of you is called *spirit*. The Romans called it your *genius* and the Greeks called it your *daimon*. Some traditions see the idea of soul as synonymous with body or with heart; others see the idea of soul as more of a universal conglomeration of all beings everywhere. Regardless of what you call it, it's the part of you that knows what wants to be lived through you. It's the part of you that has access to your inborn potential, something that James Hillman calls the "acorn theory"—the idea that your full potential is already encoded within you, just as the full potential of a mighty oak tree is encoded within a tiny acorn.[13] It's the part of you that sees this encoded potential and helps navigate you toward it.

The Mind, Heart, and Body Voices want to help keep you safe and the Soul Voice is no different. Where the Mind Voice is concerned with making life predictable and secure, the Heart Voice offers emotional feedback to help direct you, and the Body Voice does what it can to keep you vital and alive, the Soul Voice has her own thing to protect. She's in charge of protecting your inner flame, that vital source of you-ness that burns within you. The part of you that lights the fire of inspiration, the part of you that wants to grow into your own version of the majestic oak tree. She's in charge of protecting the inner flame that wants to create, grow, expand, become, and evolve.

Author Rob Bell likened this flame to a candle on a birthday cake.[14] You know how a birthday candle works—you light the candle, and as you begin to sing "Happy Birthday," you transport the cake to center stage.

13. James Hillman, *The Soul's Code: In Search of Character and Calling* (New York: Random House, 1986), 6.

14. Rob Bell, "Episode 168: The One About Boundaries," *The Robcast*. Podcast audio October 15, 2017. https://robbell.podbean.com/e/the-one-about-boundaries/

While doing so, you instinctively hold your hand near the candle to protect its flame; without your hand there, the fire can easily go out. This is how your inner flame works as well—it holds unlimited potential that can ignite your entire life on fire (just like that little birthday candle can burn the house down under the right conditions). Yet, when it's a mere flicker, it needs to be protected or else the slightest breeze can blow the flame out. The Soul Voice is like a hand protecting your inner flame, keeping your inner light safe while you travel through life.

## The Language of the Soul

The Soul uses several modalities to communicate her message. Sometimes Soul speaks in a very short sentence, just a few words at most. My favorite example of this is in the beginning of *Eat, Pray, Love*, when Elizabeth Gilbert is on her bathroom floor, awkwardly trying to have a conversation with God about whether or not she should leave her husband. The conversation turns into a prayer where she repeatedly begs for God to tell her what to do.

The answer she gets back?

*"Go back to bed, Liz."*[15]

Gilbert doesn't get a *you-should-leave* answer, nor does she get a *you-should-stay* answer. In fact, her answer had nothing to do with what she was asking. It was merely the truest thing for her to do right in that moment—go back to bed.

When the soul speaks in words, it gives answers just like Gilbert's—short sentences that don't quite seem to be the answer or clarity that you're probably hoping for. Short answers that don't exactly lay out the minutiae of how to live, but rather point you in a direction unique to that specific moment.

The Soul Voice doesn't weigh in on what you'll need to do next Tuesday, she's not concerned with how crazy you might appear, and she definitely isn't trying to impress the Joneses. From her bird's-eye point of view, she isn't concerned with making mistakes, wasting time, going the wrong di-

---

15. Elizabeth Gilbert, *Eat, Pray, Love* (New York: Penguin Books, 2006), 16.

rection, or whether or not things will work out in the way you're hoping. She accepts the chaos of life and doesn't try to micro-manage it. When she does speak, she simply offers you the next true thing to do in that moment.

The Soul Voice doesn't always communicate through cryptic short sentences. Often, she communicates messages by bringing odd things to your attention. This happened to me at my local grocery store. Typically, I'm blind to the rows of magazines that clutter the checkout stand. But, for whatever reason, that day a copy of *Sunset* magazine caught my eye—on its cover was a beautiful photograph of Big Sur.

In just a glance, right there with my carrots sliding toward the cashier, it was like I remembered who I was, who I always had been. It was like there were magnets in my bones—and they were being pulled into the picture. It was like I finally remembered something that I didn't even know I'd forgotten.

I grabbed the magazine and handed it to the cashier. I was astonished at what my hands seemed to be doing without my consent. A digital beep, and the price of the magazine showed on the screen—$11.99. Stunned at the sticker price as I expected it to be more in the three-dollar range (it had been a long time since I'd bought a magazine), I considered putting it back on the rack.

In that moment, I felt a terrible sense of free-fall—almost a sense of impending doom, or maybe intense grief. It was like the magnets in my bones had now all turned to lead. It just felt wrong, like something was very wrong. Like I was taking a very wrong turn, heading in the wrong direction. Like I'd whither up and die if I didn't buy that magazine. This made absolutely no sense to me. It was just a magazine, for God's sake. Rationally, I knew this. Rationally, I knew that magazines are on the checkout stand for this very reason—to compel you to make a purchase. But this didn't feel thoughtless or impulsive—rather, it felt like a matter of life and death. Standing at the quick-check, on an ordinary September Wednesday afternoon—a tidal wave of despair washed over me. I couldn't leave without that magazine.

Looking back now, I can see how buying that magazine set off a domino effect that radically changed the trajectory of my life. Of course, at the time I had no way of knowing why I needed to buy the magazine.

Sometimes, the soul speaks through bizarre things that will just seem to light up out of nowhere—like how the magazine stood out against the bland fluorescent-lit landscape of the grocery store. It wasn't that spotlights dropped from the ceiling, or that the magazine became sparkly and magical—but more that the magazine lit up for *me*. The scene on the cover woke up something within me.

You know how, given a full-page list of names, your eyes will almost instantly be able to find your own name within the list? The Soul Voice kind of works like that. It's like certain things, places, names, or ideas are more recognizable, easier to see, or have some sort of familiar quality to them. Almost like an invisible bell within you gets struck and pulls your attention toward that thing.

Now this doesn't mean your soul mystically floats around placing magical objects within your sight range. It works more like the list of names on a piece of paper—your name didn't miraculously appear out of nowhere, it was always there in black and white. But your name is a familiar and intimate part of your life, so you can easily and quickly filter, search, and find it on any page. Soul works in a similar way—familiar and intimate parts of your life (even when you don't seem to consciously know them yet) tend to be filtered out and lit up.

Soul Voice doesn't just communicate with you through your waking hours, she can also send you messages while you're sleeping. Throughout human history, dreams have often been correlated to divine knowledge. Different practices for dream interpretation have been passed down through stories, myths, traditions, rituals, and artifacts. Nowadays, many branches of psychology also point to the significance of dreams and their meanings. Your dreams are a rich source of soul information. They're especially helpful in times when the Soul Voice is otherwise silent, and you seem to have no other access to her.

## On the Mat: Listen to Your Soul

*Candle Meditation*

Gather any props that will help you sit comfortably—a cushion, pillow, or cozy chair—and your journal and pen. You also need a lit candle (artificial candles will not work for this exercise). Any size will do.

Find a comfortable place for this meditation. I recommend taking a few moments to honor this practice by creating a beautiful space. This meditation is about protecting your inner flame, so you may want to start by finding a space that feels sacred and protected. You might also want a blanket for extra warmth, or be near an open window if you like fresh air. You might want to quietly play music that speaks to your soul, or you might simply want silence. There's no right way to do this—every time you come to this practice, it will be unique and you'll have a different experience.

Find a safe place for your candle on the floor in front of you, on a hearth, or on an altar of some sort. Come to a comfortable seat (cross-legged, on a cushion, or in a chair) where you have a clear and close view of your candle flame. Relax and come to stillness in the pose. Lengthen your inhales and lengthen your exhales while quieting your mind. Bring your attention to the feeling of your inhale and exhale through your nostrils. Listen to the ocean-like sounds of your breath. Feel the ground beneath you, the temperature of the room, your clothes against your skin. Listen to the sounds around you, near and far. Practice paying attention to the subtle. Maybe there's a scent or a taste, maybe there's not. Check in with all five senses to help bring your awareness fully into this moment—here and now.

Bring your attention to the flame on the candle. Keep your eyes open and in a soft gaze while you meditate on the flame. Notice the quality of the flame. Maybe it's still and steady. Maybe it's erratic and busy. Keep a soft focus on the flame throughout your meditation.

Now imagine that your candle flame is the same flame within you, right in the center of your rib cage. Imagine this inner flame being your inner light, the fire that burns within your life, the spark that makes you *you*. Imagine that the flame you're observing is exactly the same as the flame within you. If the flame is still, your flame is still. If the flame is erratic, your flame is erratic. Bring your inner awareness to this light and watch it burn within you for a few cycles of breaths. When you're ready, gently lift your arms and bring your hands to your chest—one on top of the other, palms facing inward—to protect your inner flame. Imagine that your hands are sheltering and protecting it. Observe what happens to your mind, your heart, your body, and your soul while you meditate on protecting your inner flame. Spend at least five minutes in this meditation.

Ask yourself: *What does this flame want to ignite in my life?*

Journal your insights.

Now, stay with the meditation and blow your candle out. Observe the process as the remains of the flame—the heat, the smoke, the light—dissipate. Notice the smoke, the wick, the wax. Meditate on this for a few more minutes.

Ask yourself: *Where in my life is this flame most threatened?*

Journal your insights.

## Off the Mat: Listen to Your Soul

The Soul Voice is subtle. It's very difficult (almost impossible) to listen for it when you're wrapped up in your Mind Voice, when you're trying to deny your Heart Voice, and when you're ignoring your Body Voice. So before you try to incorporate Soul Voice into your daily practice, I recommend having a solid understanding of the other three voices. Once you can differentiate between each of those voices, take this Soul Voice practice out into your daily life by bringing your awareness to your relationship with your inner flame.

You can start by journaling once a day.

Ask yourself: *What does my inner flame want to ignite in my life? Where in my life is my inner flame most threatened?*

This inquiry is a powerful way to start or end the day. There's no right or wrong way to do this, nor is there any conclusive answer you might receive. It's more of a practice to take a bird's-eye view of your life, visualize that delicate flame within you, and consider what wants to be brightened, to be lit up, to be on fire in your life, and where, when, why, and by whom the flame is most threatened.

You might find that your flame is being slowly choked off every day upon entering your workplace. Or you find that your inner flame dims every time you scroll through social media. You might find that your inner flame is threatened when you lack healthy boundaries, when you're not telling the whole truth, or when you're in a state of denial; or that it shines every time you pick up a paintbrush, a book of poetry, or a packet of heirloom apple seeds. Your inner flame might come alive when you enter a public library, art museum, or greenhouse filled with orchids; and it might die a little every time you check your email, go through security at the airport, or enter a convenience store. As you move throughout your life, notice this feedback and record your insights in your journal.

The Soul Voice has preferences, just like every other voice. She lights up around certain places, certain activities, certain people. She brightens and warms in some situations and dims and sputters in others. The practice is to become aware of this inner flame within you, to separate it from the other voices and to respond to the wisdom of your Soul Voice. If Soul lights up in nature, honor this and offer her more. If she dims when watching the news, honor this and offer her less. Remember, Soul doesn't respond in a forever-way, she's simply giving feedback for that moment. Maybe next week she'll want something different, maybe tomorrow morning she'll say *yes*, where this morning she said *no*. Similar to the other voices, as you begin to listen and respond your relationship to the Soul Voice will strengthen. Eventually, this relationship will become a foundational point of inner guidance.

chapter twelve

# Allowing Soul to Guide You

How to use the soul's compass
while you're awake in the driver's seat.

Soul has a sense of place. She knows where she wants to be. She's connected to these places—a certain landscape, a park, a river, a view. Since I knew I'd be writing about Soul today, I went to one of my favorite soul spots. It's an old bookstore with a cozy coffee shop. It feels like a living room with its overstuffed couches and well-worn, dusty Persian rugs, the deep reds and blues worn thin.

This morning, I was going to sit down and write about a specific set of events tied to that *Sunset* magazine, but after about a paragraph into this chapter, I got a text from my landlord asking, "Can I call you? I need to talk to you." I am not chatty with my landlord, we have a business-only relationship, so this text was unexpected and completely out of character. I wrote back, "Yes, call me."

"There was an emergency," she said through tears. "I have to put the house up for sale tomorrow. I am sorry, I know you just moved in …"

Sometimes life interrupts our happy endings with bad news. It's like that magic trick where the tablecloth is pulled off the table and all the place settings remain undisturbed—flowers in the vase and candlesticks still intact. Except, in times like this, the spaghetti noodles are splattered across the wall, and the dishes are shattered into pieces.

Sometimes you think you know where life is leading, you think you're following your inner guidance, you think you're getting close to your destination—and then, *wham-o!*—you don't know where you are or where you're going. And you're lost all over again; the compass you held so faithfully now just slowly spins. And a new story line emerges. And you begin again.

In times like these, if you are in touch with your Soul Voice, a calm can overtake the chaos, and a quiet certainty reigns over the temporary setback. Soul doesn't worry overly much about the tiny details such as houses and cars and the clothes on your back.

I wish I could say that the Soul Voice is easy to listen to, that she points in a clear direction, that she'll guide your way flawlessly, elegantly. I wish I could say that life is controllable in that way, or predictable in that way. I wish I could say that there's a method to follow and if you do it exactly right, you'll end up with a life full of rainbows and unicorns.

But that's not how the Soul Voice works because that's not how life works.

With this news about my house, Mind is in a tailspin trying to make sense of this unpredictable, unstable life. She's busy trying to find a way to control the uncontrollable, tame the untamable. Heart is beside herself with fear, anger, confusion. Body doesn't want to leave, she doesn't want to be uprooted; she had just settled down and found her bearings.

But Soul? Since the phone call, I've been checking in with my soul. Oddly enough, she doesn't seem to care much. When I ask what she thinks, what I should do; when I beg her to tell me which way I'm supposed to go, Soul Voice has remained steadily ambiguous all day. *Warmer.* That's all I get, just a one-word answer: "Warmer."

My Soul Voice is staying pretty quiet over there in her passenger seat. She's not bothered by this news at all. She doesn't really care about the details, instability, or plans that were made. She doesn't care about my timelines or what I thought might happen.

Is it good news? Is it bad news? She doesn't have an opinion. Her job is to protect my inner flame, and other than that, I think she just loves a good story. This plot twister simply makes her smile.

She knows that I can fight for a while, if I want to. She'll wait while I argue against reality and get all freaked out. She's not in a hurry. Inevitably, she knows I'll have to surrender to life itself. So Soul sits there with her little compass and points the way forward. Not forward as in: somewhere out there. Her compass points toward a place within *me*—toward the flame in the center of my rib cage—as she whispers, *warmer*.

## Warmer

Soul's compass doesn't point to a destination, it points in the direction of a journey. *Warmer* isn't a place, it's what happens within you—your inner flame burns *warmer*—when you follow Soul's guidance. *Warmer* doesn't mean arriving at your best life, or landing somewhere as your best self. Soul's compass doesn't point toward a predetermined path that will take you to some grand arrival, nor does it point to a marvelous destination. It's not leading you to the end of a rainbow, or to a magical place where all of your dreams come true. Rather, Soul's compass leads you in the direction that fuels your inner fire, that protects your light, that stokes your brilliant flame. Her compass isn't pointing to somewhere out there, it's pointing to something within you, right here.

Soul can guide you, quite beautifully, as you journey through life—if you know how to listen to her and how to use her feedback. To listen for your Soul Voice, first shift your attention to your inner flame. If Soul's answer is *warmer*, you'll experience expansiveness in your body, heart, and mind; you might even be able to feel the warmth of your inner flame. You might feel a lightness of being, or you might feel a distinct magnets-in-your-bones pull toward a certain direction. Soul's answers tend to lean toward growth, expansion, generosity, and openness. Her answers tend to shy away from the known, regular routine; the mundane, rigid, predictable path; or from anything that might narrow, tighten, or limit you.

Don't overthink her feedback—Soul doesn't work like Mind, she's not going to speak in sentences or thoughts. She'll be a little obscure, a little vague, and often confusing. This is because she sees the whole picture, she sees your whole self. Soul Voice sees the bird's-eye view, the story, the adventure. She's not afraid and she sees you're completely capable of any challenge.

Remember, you don't have to automatically take Soul's advice. Soul is one of your Four Voices. She's a powerful voice and has a beautiful perspective to consider—but she's not the One True Voice. Sometimes Soul might say something that you're not really ready to take on. Sometimes, you might want to lean more toward your mind or your heart for a while. Nothing is wrong with this. You get to choose.

For example, let's say that *warmer* is starting a new business. This doesn't mean you need to quit your day job. It means you deal with the truth of knowing that your inner flame is being pulled toward creating something new. It means you witness yourself in your cubicle, in the meeting, on the phone, on the commute, and you notice what happens to your inner flame. You notice the magnets-in-your-bones feeling and see where Soul wants to pull you. You allow yourself to consider starting a new business, just a little bit. You acknowledge Soul and keep your eyes open for miracles, coincidences, and anything else that appears to be a soul-sign. It means you listen to your soul's advice and make tiny steps toward *warmer* while you check in with your other voices—Mind, Heart, Body—using your whole self to guide you.

Building a relationship with Soul is similar to building a relationship with any of your Four Voices. The more you listen and respond, the easier navigation becomes. Soul's advice is powerful—even if you're not ready to act on her advice. Even if you're not willing. Even if you'll never be willing. Of course, there are consequences to ignoring your Soul Voice—we'll talk about this more in the next chapter—but there are also consequences when you choose to follow her compass. Either way can be messy. Either way can be difficult. Ultimately, the choice is yours.

The important thing is to first listen to Soul, acknowledge where your inner flame might be at risk, and then decide if, how, or when you want to take action. Soul will wait, she's patient and she sees the entire picture. She's not attached to an outcome, she's just doing what she can to protect your flame. Give Soul the opportunity to speak, voice her opinion, and point you toward *warmer*—this, even without taking her advice, is incredibly powerful.

## Magic 8-Ball

It's easy to misunderstand, misread, or misinterpret Soul's compass. If you don't understand what *warmer* really means, Soul's guidance seems about as reliable as a plastic Magic 8-Ball. I remember shaking that ball at twelve years old, trying to hold my question in my mind as if my entire destiny relied solely on my ability to focus.

"Am I going to marry Charlie?"

I turned the ball over and waited for the die to center in the blue liquid. "My sources say no," it said.

I shook the ball and asked again, burning with the same question. "Will I marry Charlie?" This time I closed my eyes, as if the Magic 8-Ball had punished me for peeking.

"Reply hazy, try again," it said. I shook that damned ball over and over, repeatedly asking the same question, hoping that eventually I'd get the answer I was looking for: "It is decidedly so."

Yep, sometimes trying to listen to your Soul Voice feels a lot like that. The feedback shows up as nonsensical, erratic, ambiguous gibberish. As you move through your life, you might not be able to see the big picture. You might not be able to see the entire story from start to finish. Check in with your soul, have a dialogue with her just as you would with any of the Four Voices. Ask her for guidance, for advice. Home in on her compass and see if you can orient yourself toward *warmer*. If you're getting what feels like a Magic 8-Ball answer, don't be alarmed. Change your focus to your inner flame, notice if this changes the way you ask the question, or the way you might need to navigate. And then, ask again.

For example, you might be wondering if you should train for a marathon. Soul may come up with a Magic 8-Ball answer like, "Hmmm, maybe?" And this can be frustrating, because you might really want to know the answer. You might ask and ask, but never get a good soul-read. Unfortunately, Soul won't be too bothered by your sense of urgency.

If you're not clear on an answer, I suggest aligning your question with your inner flame. In the marathon example, the Soul Voice's feedback really depends on what the marathon means to you. If it isn't a soul-inner-fire thing, keep digging. Try to follow *warmer* until you find something that lights up. Maybe you'll start by asking about a marathon, but as you dig deeper, you might realize you really just want to be outdoors for a few hours a day. Then you might start spending a few hours outdoors and you might really wish you had a sketch pad and pencils with you. And then you might decide to take an art class.

Magic 8-Ball readings just mean you need to keep going, keep digging, keep searching. Eventually, you'll find something that sparks, or pulls—something that has its own sense of gravity. Then step in that direction, stay aware of your inner light, watch for signs of *warmer,* and step by step, Soul will show you the way.

## Toto Effect

There's one more thing about Soul that you need to know. As I said earlier, she loves a good story. Your soul isn't bent in the same direction as your other voices. She's not focused on keeping life predictable, safe, or secure. She doesn't argue with reality and she's not trying to make the universe behave. She's not in a hurry and she's not married to an outcome. She lives in the moment, yet her perspective is timeless.

She sees you as stronger, smarter, and more capable than you will probably ever see yourself. And, unlike you, she's not afraid. She loves a good adventure. She simply smiles and says, *Bring it.*

Which is why Soul often turns your entire world upside down.

I call this the Toto Effect—after Dorothy's Toto in the *Wizard of Oz.* For the sake of simplicity, I'll keep my analogy focused on the movie rather than the book. You've probably seen the movie a hundred times, but to really get a feel for the Toto Effect, I suggest watching just once while focusing only on Toto. You'll see that throughout the film, Toto steers the story. He starts the adventure by biting Miss Gulch. To protect her little dog, Dorothy runs away. This is why she gets caught in the tornado that takes her to Oz. Without Toto, there would be no Oz. Toto is the first to fall asleep in the field of poppies, and he is the one who pulls back the curtain to reveal the true identity of the Great and Powerful Wizard. Even in the last few moments of the story, when the Wizard is about to escort Dorothy back to Kansas in his hot air balloon, Toto sees a pretty little blue-eyed cat and jumps out of the basket to chase her. Without Toto, Dorothy would have been returned home by an iconic father figure, rather than learning that the very shoes she'd been walking on had held the power to bring her home all along.

Soul can be a lot like Toto. Soul loves the story but she's also your trusted companion. She protects you and you protect her. Sometimes she bites Miss Gulch and you end up getting stuck in a tornado. Other times she jumps out of the basket at the last minute and forces you to rely on your ruby slippers to get you home. She not only drives the story of your life forward, but also makes choices that kindle your inner flame, making sure that you keep burning bright.

In the moment, it can feel terrible when your little dog jumps out of the basket and you think you've lost your chance to get home. Often, the Toto Effect feels awful and confusing and upsetting at first. But when you look at your history, and look at the landmarks and turning points of your life—those times when you thought you'd turn left but at the last minute you turned right—those moments may have been the Toto Effect in action. When something sudden, major, or unexpected happens, instead of falling apart, keep one eye open to see if this might be Soul jumping out of the basket, biting Miss Gulch, or pulling back the curtain on the Wizard.

This whole phone call out of the blue about my house might be a Toto Effect. I'm not saying that my wild little Soul caused this. I'm saying that Soul has a bigger view of the story—maybe she saw this coming? Maybe she didn't. Maybe this phone call will be the reason why I end up buying a home and living in this town for the next forty years. Maybe the phone call will inspire me to find a different house—one I didn't even know I wanted. Maybe it will take me to a place where I can put down roots. Or maybe, I'll discover that I also love a good adventure and that I'd rather travel. Or maybe, nothing will happen at all—and I'll stay right here, just like I'd originally planned.

Who knows? It's too soon to tell.

But when I look at the phone call as a Toto Effect, I begin to see wide-open possibilities in front of me. Instead of being tunneled down into my little life, my creativity has been sparked, my inner flame has started burning brighter, and I have begun dreaming about a new horizon. My plan about buying a home in a few years might be something I act on next week. My dream about packing everything up and living out of an Airstream while traveling the country? That might happen, too. Life is big and so are you. And the story is nowhere near finished.

## On the Mat: Move toward Warmer

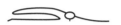

### Child's Pose—Balasana

Begin in Child's Pose and turn your awareness inward. Allow all tension in your shoulders, arms, and neck to drain away. Keep your gaze drawn inward with your eyes closed.

Child's Pose is an introspective pose. Your strong backbone protects you while you curl your awareness into your center. Bring your attention to your inner flame and imagine that this pose is protecting your inner flame. Spend at least three minutes relaxing into this pose, continuing with your conscious breath. As you draw yourself deeper into the pose, and deeper into the inquiry, keep your inner awareness open to your Soul Voice.

Ask yourself: *What makes my inner light burn warmer? What does my soul truly desire?*

Notice any pictures, memories, dreams, or ideas that come to mind. Notice any people, relationships, or places that come to mind. Notice any actions that might need to be taken, or any changes that may need to be made to honor Soul's feedback. Remain open and simply listen without reaction. Record your observations in your journal.

Repeat the process several times. Drop into Child's Pose and bring your attention to your inner light. Continue with the inquiry practice and record your insights. You may discover that each round takes you to deeper layers of soul desires. You may discover that your Soul Voice offers the same answer again and again. There's no right way to do this practice. Simply curl into yourself, hold the pose, and dialogue with your Soul Voice.

Soul will guide you if you let her. She'll lead you through mysteries and adventures. She'll open doors and light up things that were previously concealed. Your job is to simply take the next small step along that soul-lit path.

## Off the Mat: Move toward Warmer

Whether you're on the mat or off, listening for your soul's desires has the power to shape your day, your week, your life. Regardless of where you are, or what's happening around you, you have the ability to drop in and dialogue with your Soul Voice. For fifteen years, I've worked with students privately, in retreats, in workshops, and in online courses. Out of all the questions I offer, the number one question, the one that seems to pack the most punch, the one that seems to be the most commonly overlooked is: *What do you want?*

This question never fails to draw a silent, unexpected pause. Because the truth is, most of my students are busy thinking about what's happening. They're occupied with reacting to the events of the day. They take out the trash, answer their emails, make lunches, and do errands. I'm no different—it's easy to forget who you really are, to forget the sacred nature of your life. Often, my students can easily reel off a laundry list of things they don't want. But when I ask them, "What makes your inner light burn warmer? What does your soul truly desire?" they draw a blank, they have no idea.

So, I urge you to ask. I urge you to ask yourself this question every single day. Stay in dialogue with Soul.

Ask yourself: *What makes my inner light burn warmer? What does my soul truly desire?*

Soul is brave. Like Toto, she runs ahead and you have no choice but to follow. When you listen with a curious mind, an open heart, and a steady body, the soul's confusing instructions won't startle you. You'll make that phone call, tender your resignation, buy that bus ticket. Body, Heart, and Mind tend to soften when Soul speaks. They stop their worry chatter and a beautiful stillness opens within you. Soul speaks within that stillness and shows you the way forward.

# chapter thirteen

# Dark Night of the Soul

How to chart your course
when you can't access Soul's compass.

I think that anything you love deeply will eventually break your heart. There's no way around it. To love is to be devastated by the giving of yourself to that person, that calling, that place. Whether it's parenthood, a career, a place, a marriage, to truly give yourself over to a relationship means that you surrender the safety of separateness. It's where there is no longer a me and a you, only an us. And in that us, you risk yourself for all the beauty and all the ruin ahead.

The dark night of any soul doesn't happen quickly, nor does it happen suddenly. Your eyes adjust as the light slowly dims. It happens so gradually you don't even realize until it's too late—until you're standing in complete darkness with no inner flame to light your path. This moment of darkness is a threshold, a place to pass through not because it's a test or a measurement of your strength but more because it is part of the process of living, loving, of being loved. To walk through this threshold means you have to surrender everything—and I mean everything—about who you think you are and what you think you believe. It doesn't mean you stand there and wait until you find the light again; it means you surrender everything that brought you to this moment. And without light, without any remaining beliefs, without any remaining faith, you make yourself take the next step into that black night.

Sometimes, this is how wayfinding work goes. Sometimes, you have to lose everything. And then from rock bottom, you begin to find your way home.

The dark night of the soul isn't necessarily brought on by deep grief or terrible losses. Sometimes it's caused by living a life you don't love for too long. Sometimes it's caused by chasing the wrong thing only to arrive at a destination that's utterly empty. And sometimes it happens when everything you thought to be true is, tragically, just an illusion. No matter what brings you to this place, you'll know it's the dark night of your soul because you won't be able to rely on the light of your inner flame. It's here you must learn to completely surrender. It's here you learn to walk in the dark.

During a period I would call the dark night of my soul, the grief was debilitating. In one way, I was more present in my life than I'd ever been. The hustle had been knocked out of me. I had been taken to my knees, humbled. All I could do was simply make it through the day. And then to try to endure the night.

The nights during that time were long. Coyotes cackled like a coven of witches out there in the darkness beyond and woke me up at one o'clock. Then again at three. I'd wake up at four, not knowing how I was going to get through the miles of hours before I could go to bed again. My body was exhausted, but I couldn't sleep. All I could do was wait. Wait through the night, wait for the day to break. Wait for it to get dark once again.

I couldn't make sense out of my life. Out of my career. Out of my work. Out of love. I'd pull out my yoga mat, thinking that I'd find solace there. I can't tell you how many times I did this—twenty, thirty?—I'd lay out my dusty mat, and go through the motions. I'd try to invoke the mystic, the mystery. Nothing. I'd light my candles, chant my mantras, and put together the perfect playlist. Nothing. I couldn't find any spark that would light my inner flame.

The only thing I could do was wake up, drive my daughter to school, and then lie on the couch until I did the routine in reverse—pick her up from school, drive home, and go back to bed. I watched a lot of TV. I read a lot of books.

I did this for months.

Calling it the dark "night" of the soul seems to be a misnomer. For most of us, it's more like a dark year of the soul. And, just as your light doesn't completely vanquish in an instant—it won't begin to shine again all at once. Think of the dark night more like an eclipse of your inner flame—where life's shadow obscures what's within you. Where it might take a long time for the light to regain its full strength.

## When the Flame Goes Out

You can't force your inner flame to burn. Fire needs air, it needs fuel, it needs space. The minute you try to control it, contain it, smother it, it'll vanquish. Although these moments of darkness are terrible, painful, and heartbreaking, they are inevitable. For if you give yourself to any journey wholeheartedly, you will eventually have to cross territory without a way to light your path.

When the flame goes out, it means you've come to the end of the road. And the path you took to get there will not be the path you must take to leave. Whatever your beliefs, whatever your attachments, whatever you think you loved about your original path, it will all have to be surrendered, left behind, and grieved.

To walk in the dark, you must be willing to know nothing. You must be willing to be wrong. You must be willing to surrender. Most importantly, though, you must walk. Sure, you can rest for a while. You can lie on your couch, watch TV, and lick your wounds for a week, a month, a year. But eventually, you'll have to step out into that black water of the night, into the unknown depths. And instead of guiding yourself by the light of your inner flame, you'll have to guide yourself by starlight, by moon shadow, or simply by touch alone. You'll have to take a step into nothingness. And then another. And you'll have to keep taking those steps until finally, once you've entered a new place, something unexpectedly sparks within you. And you'll find your flame burning again. But this time, the flame will be different. This time, it will be stronger.

## The Witness

In those moments of the dark night, I don't think Soul ever forsakes you. I don't think she ever loses her way. Nor do I think she ever leaves your side. Even in times where your inner flame has gone completely dark, I believe that Soul sits vigil, waiting. During those hours, those years, you may only be able to rely on your three other voices. While walking in the dark, you may have to steer only with Mind, Heart, and Body. But that doesn't mean Soul has left the passenger seat. It simply means she's silent, waiting, watching.

Soul's compass points toward *warmer*, toward what makes your inner flame burn warmer. Her compass does not have a *colder* reading. When you steer your life away from *warmer*, Soul's compass can no longer guide you—it just spins. When you continue marching toward *colder*, you'll get no feedback from Soul. That was my great mistake. I thought that eventually, if I continued on, Soul would chime in. I projected my old beliefs onto Soul—thinking that I needed to suffer, work hard, sacrifice, and that in the end, I'd find access to my Soul Voice. I thought that if I just kept going down a road called *Colder*, I'd eventually hit a town called *Warmer*. But no matter how far down that cold road you go, it never leads you to *warmer*. And eventually, you'll have to turn around, give up, and take a different road.

Soul's compass requires movement; when you stay still, you get no feedback. You could be one inch away from the target, but if you refuse to budge, there will only be silence. Soul can guide you beautifully, but she requires that you take a step. If you feel paralyzed, scared, unsure, or doubtful, take a step anyway. All it takes is one tiny action toward what might protect your inner flame. If you step toward *warmer*, you'll get feedback. Maybe it'll feel like that magnets-in-your-bones feeling, or maybe you'll see soul-signs, coincidences that seem to light up pathways you hadn't seen before. If you get no feedback, take a step in a different direction.

In the dark times, Soul is your witness. She quietly holds her compass, watching for the needle to move. She sees the bird's-eye perspective of your life. She sees the path that led you to this moment, and sees the way you must take to walk out of the darkness. She loves a good story and knows that every great story has a beginning, a middle, an end. She's not attached to an outcome, she's not attached to any particular Point B. She's in charge of protecting your flame, but she also knows that she can't light the flame for you. She can only throw a spark in your direction. And if you're watching, listening, waiting, responding, that spark just might catch fire. And when it does, Soul will point toward the flame in the middle of your rib cage and whisper, "*Warmer.*"

## Finding Your Way in the Dark

If you've found yourself in the dark and cannot find a way out, please know there have been countless others here before you. There are countless others with you. And there will be countless more to come. To endure the dark night of the soul is to be human. For centuries, poets, mystics, and spiritual teachers have taught about how to find your way through this particular darkness. If you're stuck and want some guidance, these are a few of the things that I've found helpful:

### Pay Attention to Your Dreams

Keep a journal or notebook by your bed and jot down anything you remember upon waking, even if it's just one or two words. Sometimes, when you have no access to Soul Voice in the day, she'll speak to you through dreams at night. Remember that dreams are symbolic; the people, objects, and situations in your dreams are not to be taken literally. Instead, jot down what you remember, ask yourself what feeling comes up when you think about the dream. Notice if that feeling matches anything in your present-day life. Look at your dreams as your Soul Voice trying to speak. What is she trying to say? Where might she be guiding you?

### Read Poetry

Poetry has been a light for me during my darkest hours. You don't have to be a literary scholar to benefit from poetry. A good poem works on you— you don't have to work on it. Just let the words wash through you, like you're listening to a song. The more you listen, the more you'll hear.

*Look to Mythology*

Mythology is rich and its stories can steer you. Whether you're looking to Hindu, Greek, Roman, or Native American mythology, no matter what the story, or where in the world it originated, mythology holds within it ancient archetypes, and your soul recognizes these motifs. Many myths are intended for the very purpose of helping one through the dark night.

Joseph Campbell, who devoted his entire life to the study of mythology, taught that myths serve four major functions. First, there's a mystical function, bringing your focus to the wonder of the universe, and the mystery of who you are. Second, myths bring mystery to science—giving it a deeper and richer meaning. Third, myths help integrate social order, giving societies a common belief system. But he says, there is a fourth function of mythology and that is the pedagogical function, of how to live a human lifetime under any circumstances.[16] Myths can teach you how to live a human life—even in darkness.

*Go Out into Nature*

Nature is neutral and no matter how dark life gets, nature can be a compassionate witness through your journey. Observe nature, experience it, breathe it in. When you look closely, you'll see all the small miracles and terrible hardships within it. You'll see the struggle to simply stay alive and you'll see the unexpected beauty that unfolds even in the humblest of places. When life goes dark, and you can no longer hear your soul, go out into the wild. Listen to the wind, watch the stars, listen for the birds. Take your shoes off and touch the dirt. Sit and wait. The ocean will rise and will then fall away. The birds will return to their nests. Trees will grow tall and lose their leaves. Even the flowers will fade and their seeds will give way to new life. The cycle of birth and death is throughout nature, in every corner. When you've lost your way in the darkness, sit still and let nature guide you.

16. Joseph Campbell, *Occidental Mythology* (New York: Penguin, 1991), 519–522.

### Study Spiritual Texts

If you've lost your way, consider returning to ancient wisdom. There's a reason why books such as the Bible, the Quran, the Tao Te Ching, and Patanjali's Yoga Sutra are in still print centuries after they were originally written—they are still relevant. Scriptures and sutra comfort me, reminding me that I'm not the first one to feel lost in the darkness, and I won't be the last. There's not one right way out of the dark night of the soul; there are many.

### Participate in Ritual and Ceremony

Ritual is mythology in action. It's a full-body participation in the story. There's something mysterious that unlocks between you and your soul when you participate in ritual. Whether it's attending a graduation, wedding, funeral, or maybe even a morning Mass, these social rituals help put life into perspective. In yoga, the ritual of chanting *om*, or of saying *namaste* at the end of a yoga class seal the practice and help you touch on the greater meaning behind your actions. If you want, try a ritual at home: kneel, place your hands together in prayer, and bow your head. This is mythology in action. This powerful ritual invokes the sacred, the mystery, and the nature of inquiry. It invokes the art of asking and the art of listening.

## Full Circle

I always thought that at the end of the dark night of the soul there'd be a grand sense of homecoming. Maybe another round of heartbreak, or an overwhelming relief at finding an inkling of light kindling within. I thought it might feel sacred or even holy. But that's not what I've found to be true.

Instead, it's more like coming full circle. Back to where you started. Back to who you've always been. Except this time, you no longer believe the old stories and you're no longer chasing the foolish illusions. This time you're not longing for some far-off destination. Rather, you're content to journey right into the center of your own self.

After shedding everything that the dark night requires, you won't find yourself in a brand new life. Instead, you'll find yourself in the life that's been available to you all along. No longer searching for a destination, you allow the adventure to come alive from within you.

To everyone around you, you may look exactly as you've always appeared. But you will know the truth. You will know the difference. Through seasoned eyes, you will see everything—your loved ones, your life, yourself—with more generosity. Refined by experience, you'll find an unexpected beauty in the simplest of things.

Maybe you'll find a sense of serenity as you chop vegetables for dinner. Or you'll find yourself smiling while standing in line at the post office. Or you'll find an unexpected beauty within the busyness of your daily tasks—while taking your kids to school, washing the dishes, or rolling out your mat at your Tuesday evening yoga class. This unexpected calm, this unexpected familiarity, this unexpected everyday-ness of just being here; this is the glorious homecoming. This is the destination. This is yoga.

## On the Mat: Trust the Darkness

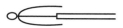

*Savasana*

Lie down on your back. Stretch your legs long and allow your arms to fall by your side. Allow yourself to take up space. Allow yourself to rest. Savasana—Corpse Pose—is a ritual. In Savasana, you not only lie down to enact your death, you also allow yourself to let go, to rest, and to physically, spiritually, and emotionally experience the dark night of the soul. Savasana can teach you about grief; the physical pose teaches you what surrender feels like. It also teaches you that as you let go completely, you are held. The floor holds you. The ground holds you.

This is a full-body experience of the dark night of the soul. You allow yourself to completely surrender, having given yourself wholeheartedly to the practice. You allow every muscle to relax, you allow all Four Voices to silence. And then, you are simply held. The ground holds you, as it always has, as it always will. No matter what you think you've lost, no matter what you want to keep, eventually all roads lead to this ground. Eventually, all roads lead to Savasana.

## Off the Mat: Trust the Darkness

In moments when you feel completely lost, moments when you feel for-
saken, forgotten, or alone, come to the ground and lie down in Savasana.
The ground is a powerful teacher. In class, Savasana is a beautiful ritual that
helps you to reset and renew. Off the mat, Savasana is a full-body practice
of allowing yourself to be held. The ground knows where you are. It knows
how to hold you. When you lie on the ground, the entire floor holds your
weight. When you lie on the floor, gravity holds you in place. Let yourself
be held. Let yourself surrender. Let yourself be found.

# Wayfinding with Your Soul Voice

Soul communicates in mysterious ways, sometimes through a still small voice, sometimes by lighting things up, and sometimes through a feeling of magnets in your bones, as if something has its own sense of gravity. Soul watches over your inner flame and offers feedback that helps to not only protect that flame, but also to kindle the flame warmer. The practice of inquiry—the art of asking questions—helps you to clarify the soul's message, and determine the advice or direction that the voice offers you. As you work through Soul Inquiry, keep your focus on the bird's-eye view, on your inner flame, and on the part of you that's timeless. There's no right way to listen to Soul Voice. The work here is to stay present while you bring your attention to your inner light.

## Soul Inquiry Method

*Set an intention to have a conversation with your soul.*
Imagine having a conversation with someone who sees the bird's-eye view of your life. Imagine that you can open a dialogue with the timeless part of you—the protector of your inner flame. By setting an intention, you focus your attention on receiving your soul's wisdom. Do not overthink things, there is no right or wrong way to do this. Do your best to stay aware of your inner flame throughout this inquiry practice. Be gentle and patient—take it

slow and observe the subtle. Simply state to yourself—out loud or in your head—*I intend to have a conversation with my soul.*

### Look for Soul signs—symbolic or metaphorical messages.

Take a full inventory of any interesting coincidences, anything that has suddenly "lit up" for you, any moments of déjà vu, any strange dreams, or any interesting doors that have seemed to open for you lately. Record any images, insights, or ideas that come to you. Take a full inventory of any Toto Effect possibilities, or any information that may feel like a Magic 8-Ball Soul response. You may not have any immediate Soul signs that come to mind. That's okay. The primary purpose of this inquiry process is to set the intention of opening a dialogue with the Soul Voice so that you become more adept at listening to its cues. Soul signs may or may not give you feedback on the particular situation in question, but it is still important to note them. The more you become attuned to all of the potential messages of your soul, the better you will become at checking in with the Soul Voice on a regular basis.

### What's the situation?

Now, you can move on to checking in with your soul for navigation. Whether you're wanting to clarify a difficult situation, get to your version of Point B, make a decision, or find your way when you're entirely lost—start with articulating your situation. In just a sentence or two, write a short version of your dilemma, quandary, or story.

### Regarding this situation, is your inner flame being threatened? If so, how?

Consider all aspects of this situation from a bird's-eye point of view and see how the larger picture of this situation fits into your life overall. From this point of view, consider whether the situation endangers or threatens your inner flame—that vital source of you-ness that burns within you. Consider whether this situation threatens the part of you that lights the fire of inspiration, the part of you that wants to create, grow, expand, become, and evolve. If yes, take some time to articulate the way(s) in which it is threatened, or under what specific conditions your inner flame might come to be threatened in this situation.

### Regarding this situation, what action would make your inner flame burn warmer?

Soul's compass points in the direction of a journey. Your inner flame burns warmer when you follow Soul's guidance. Considering this situation, Soul's compass points in a direction that fuels your inner fire, protects your light, and stokes your brilliant flame. Determine what small action would be a step toward *warmer* here.

### Specify your Point B for this particular situation.

Think about the big picture here and articulate your larger intention, focus, commitment, and priority.

### Is Soul's advice taking you to where you want to go?

Reflect on the information that you've received from your Soul Voice. Reflect on what feels warmer, and what action needs to be taken to protect your inner flame. Sometimes Soul won't necessarily direct you to your specific Point B. And that's okay. This might mean that your soul has a different journey in mind. Remember, you do not have to take Soul's advice, her voice is simply one voice to listen to. To guide with your whole self, you want to consider all Four Voices before determining your path.

### What can you do to honor your soul's wisdom as you journey to Point B?

Whether or not you take Soul's advice, determine how you might honor your soul's wisdom by protecting your inner flame. This might mean that you offer your soul nourishment in ways that have nothing to do with this particular situation. Maybe you offer your soul more creativity, more time for ritual, more time for contemplation. Maybe you simply move forward on your path with eyes-wide-open attention on your inner flame. Consider how you might honor your relationship to your soul as you move forward.

*Thank Soul.*

Here's your new script: "Thank you Soul for trying to protect my inner flame. I will do my best to honor your input. My larger intention, focus, commitment, and priority is _____. I will stay connected to your wisdom as I move in that direction."

# Quick Review of the Soul Inquiry Method

1. Set an intention to have a conversation with your soul.

2. Look for Soul signs—symbolic or metaphorical messages.

3. What's the situation?

4. Regarding this situation, is your inner flame being threatened? If so, how?

5. Regarding this situation, what action would make your inner flame burn warmer?

6. Specify your Point B for this particular situation.

7. Is Soul's advice taking you to where you want to go?

8. What can you do to honor your soul's wisdom as you journey to Point B?

9. Thank Soul. Here's your new script: "Thank you Soul for trying to protect my inner flame. I will do my best to honor your input. My larger intention, focus, commitment, and priority is _____.
I will stay connected to your wisdom as I move in that direction."

## *Example: House Is Up for Sale*

**1. Set an intention to have a conversation with your soul.**

**2. Look for Soul signs—symbolic or metaphorical messages.** I got a phone call from my landlord letting me know that she's listing my house for sale. Soul-sign seems to be about the impermanence of the specific house I live in.

**3. What's the situation?** My house has just been listed for sale and I'm not sure what to do.

4. **Regarding this situation, is your inner flame being threatened? If so, how?** No, my flame isn't being threatened. As long as I continue to believe that I am worthy of living in a beautiful home, of being loved, and of having stability—I think I'll be fine.

5. **Regarding this situation, what action would make your inner flame burn warmer?** The only actions that feels warmer is to simply wait. Even though my other voices want to fight reality or try to control the outcome, my Soul Voice seems to want me to just be patient.

6. **Specify your Point B for this particular situation.** To live a happy, full, and whole life with my daughter, and to make sure she can continue her educational pursuits.

7. **Is Soul's advice taking you to where you want to go?** I have several options moving forward that will protect my daughter's education, her pursuits, and also protect our life together. So, yes, I think that Soul's advice of just being patient is in line with my overall Point B.

8. **What can you do to honor your soul's wisdom as you journey to Point B?** I will continue to check in with Soul Voice on a regular basis. Her message might change as time goes on, for now, patience seems to be the overall message.

9. **Thank Soul.** Here's your new script: "Thank you Soul for trying to protect my inner flame. I will do my best to honor your input. My larger intention, focus, commitment, and priority is to live a happy, full, and whole life with my daughter, and to make sure she can continue her educational pursuits. I will stay connected to your wisdom as I move in that direction."

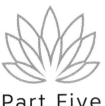

## Part Five
# Bringing the Four Voices Together

By bringing together all Four Voices—Mind, Heart, Body, and Soul—you have access to the wisdom of your whole self. By eliminating the clutter of the mind, following the feedback offered through your emotions, caring for the animal of your body, and honoring your inner flame, you're able to use your inner maps and compass for reliable guidance. As we move through the next section, you'll learn how to navigate using the wisdom of all Four Voices.

# chapter fourteen

# The Four Voices

How to find your way with all Four Voices.

Wayfinding using all Four Voices requires a firm grip on your steering wheel. It means that, from the driver's seat, you're able to listen to the Mind Voice, clear the clutter, and find the truth. It means that you're able to check in with your Heart Voice, determine the quality of emotion present, and take action based on the emotion's feedback. It means that you're connected to the animal of your body, that you're able to consider its instinctual wisdom and honor the physical sensations present. These three voices offer you the map, the minute-by-minute guidance that you need for any terrain.

This doesn't mean that they agree, nor does it mean that their navigation points to a consistent route. While awake at the wheel, you have to remember that you are the adult, you are in charge, you are ultimately the wayfinder. From this perspective, you can have compassion for Mind, who's trying to make things predictable and safe. You can discern whether Heart is reacting to Mind's narrative or if she's offering you a way forward. You can take care of Body and home in on the subtle wisdom she offers. From the driver's seat, you determine your way forward knowing that the three voices in the backseat are all trying to protect you in their own way.

If Mind says, "Go left," and Heart and Body say, "Go right," you must choose which voice to listen to. This means that you'll need the bird's-eye viewpoint offered by Soul as well as a clear understanding of where you're trying to get to: your Point B.

Start with asking the Four Voices a small question. The more specific, the better. It's best to practice charting your course with small and seemingly insignificant questions, rather than immediately jumping into the tough life-altering questions. Maybe you start with asking the Four Voices, "What do I want to wear today?" or "Should I go to yoga tonight?" or "Should I take the dog for a walk?"

As an example, let's look at the yoga question. You'll ask Mind, Heart, Body, and Soul to answer the question.

You begin by asking Mind the question: "Should I go to yoga tonight?" Mind might say, "Yes, you need to do this, you made a promise to yourself. You're going to feel bad if you don't go. And what will people think if you just go home and relax on the couch tonight? But, it was such a long day today, and it would be so nice to just go home after work." As the driver, you have to cut through the mind's clutter. Mind offers ambiguous answers. Sometimes Mind even argues with herself. Often, she'll say yes *and* she'll say no. This is normal, and this is also why it's important to listen to all Four Voices before you decide on your direction. In general, you'll need to be able to allow Mind to speak, without reacting to her opinions.

Next, you'll check what your heart offers. For the question of going to yoga tonight, you'll need to imagine yourself on each side of the answer. Imagine going to yoga. What emotions come up? Then imagine not going to yoga. What emotions come up? You might imagine going to yoga and feelings of stress or anxiety arise—these are emotions from the fear family that mean *run* from danger. Then you might imagine not going to yoga and immediately feel a sense of peace. As the driver, this would be interpreted as the heart saying no to yoga. On the flip side, you may imagine going to class and feel peace, and the idea of missing class might bring up a feeling of sadness—an emotion that means the loss of something important. This would be interpreted as the heart saying yes to yoga. For the sake of the example, let's say that you receive a no answer from your Heart Voice. Remember, this is merely feedback from one voice for one particular day. This doesn't mean that your heart is forever against going to yoga. Rather, this is about checking in with Heart and allowing her to weigh in. From the driver's seat, you listen to her feedback and then move on to the other voices before determining your course.

Once you have clarity on Heart's message, you'll check in with Body. Consider both sides of the equation—as you did with Heart—and watch for subtle physical cues. Imagine going to yoga tonight and see if your body relaxes or tightens. Imagine not going to class tonight and see if your body relaxes or tightens. This is subtle feedback and it will not be scripted in words. Be aware that your Mind Voice may want to hijack this conversation. The more rules and judgments you have about the particular topic, the more the mind will try to pose as a different voice. So go gently and watch for anything that resembles words or thoughts. The minute you're internally hearing a voice say something like, "I think I feel fill-in-the-blank" (keyword: *think*), that's your mind trying to impersonate another voice— Heart, Body, or Soul. Thank Mind for trying to keep you safe, and then ask the original voice again. In this example, you'd check in with Body again, remembering that the information comes from the animal, not from the cerebral part of you. The animal part of you might relax when you imagine being at yoga, or it might relax when you imagine staying home. For the sake of this example, let's say the animal relaxes when you imagine going to yoga. That would be a Body Voice yes to going to yoga.

Lastly, you'll check in with Soul. You can simply ask Soul, "Do you want to go to yoga tonight?" and you might instantly feel a magnets-in-your-bones answer. You may also just get a one-word response from Soul—no or yes. If you're unclear about Soul's answer, look at the question from an inner-flame standpoint to determine if going to yoga protects your inner flame, or threatens your inner flame. In this example, let's say your soul knows that yoga protects your inner flame. Soul's answer is yes.

In this example of going to yoga tonight, the Four Voices do not agree. This is often where you'll find yourself with wayfinding. Your mind and heart may say no while your body and soul say yes. This is where, as the driver, you must choose which voice to listen to. This is where, as the driver, you chart your course.

You can choose to go forward listening to your mind and heart. Or you can choose to go forward listening to your body and soul. There is no "correct" voice to listen to, nor is there a "best" way forward. There's simply, you, the driver, making a choice to take a left or a right. This isn't a forever choice, it's just one of many choices as you move through your life.

Consider your Point B and which of the voices seem to align with your desired destination. This is where you get to decide what type of life you want to live and what kind of journey you wish to make. Ideally, you'd love for all Four Voices to align, so that there's one clear path ahead. But that's not the way wayfinding works.

Wayfinding isn't a science, it's an art. There are thousands of roads you can take to your Point B. There's no right way, nor are there shortcuts. Wayfinding means you listen for the subtle cues being offered from all Four Voices and you do your best to move in the direction that feels right for you in the moment. It means you stay open to feedback so that you're able to adjust when you go off course, hit a dead end, or just keep going in circles.

This doesn't mean that you have to be 100 percent eyes-wide-open and connected all of the time. Wayfinding doesn't require perfection. Rather, it means you chart a path, and when things start to look a little unfamiliar, or you start feeling a bit ungrounded, you check in again. It means that anytime you find yourself asleep in the backseat, you regain consciousness, move yourself to the front seat, and begin to drive your life again. Rather than finding yourself on a straight line, you'll find yourself zig-zagging through life. Yet, no matter where you zig or where you zag, you'll be able to recognize the landmarks, become familiar with the terrain, and eventually know how to get yourself home.

As you practice your skills, you'll get better at reading the nuances of your inner voices. You'll become more aware of your patterns, and you'll have a better understanding of which voices tend to offer you the best information. Eventually, you'll be able to stand in any moment and quickly ask yourself, "What does Mind want? What does Heart want? What does Body want? What does Soul want?" You'll be able to discount the mind's desire to control, you'll understand the messages embedded in your emotions, the physical feedback offered by your body, and you'll have a strong sense of your soul's compass. When you are connected to your inner guidance, no matter what life throws at you or where you find yourself, you'll always be able to find your way.

# Wayfinding with Your Four Voices

## Four Voices Inquiry Method

*What's one small thing you'd like to understand or get clear about?*

Start with something small. Every big situation is made up of hundreds of smaller pieces. The Four Voices are clearest when you work on the small parts. This practice is about navigating the Four Voices and listening for the distinct feedback that each voice offers. Write it down.

*What does your Mind Voice say about this?*

The Mind Voice is the thinking center, the inner critic, the judge. This voice speaks in words, sentences, and questions. It can often sound critical, fearful, and controlling. It often sounds like old scripts from childhood or damaging statements from authority figures. It often asks a bunch of point-less questions meant to shame and control you into behaving.

*What does your Heart Voice say about this?*

The Heart Voice speaks in emotions and offers emotional guidance. An emotion is an internal physical response that shows you how you truthfully feel about something. The work is to stay present while you feel your feel-ings, to use your heart and emotions as a navigation system and to become conscious of your habits associated with avoiding your feelings. Your heart, the center of your emotions, offers you critical information in real time.

Although certain emotions might be more dominant, they do not stand alone. In every situation, fear, shame, guilt, anger, and sadness should also be considered.

### What does your Body Voice say about this?

The Body Voice comes from the animal of your body; it reacts with instincts. It holds your history and memories in physical form. This voice speaks in animalistic instincts and reactions. When this voice is ignored, it often resorts to physical pain, discomfort, or ailments to get your attention.

### What does your Soul Voice say about this?

The Soul Voice is your higher consciousness; the protector of your inner flame. It offers kind and wise guidance. By leaning away from the ticker tape of your mind, opening your heart and being willing to feel the entire spectrum of feelings, and by building trust with the animal of your body, you open up a connection with your Soul Voice. This voice speaks quietly in very few words. Sometimes it's easier to access this voice if you imagine what your soul would say to a small child. This voice is always kind.

### Specify your Point B for this particular situation

Think about the big picture here and articulate your larger intention, focus, commitment, and priority.

### Given the feedback of all Four Voices, what feels like the truest course of action for you to take at this time?

Remember that no single voice should hold the authority; the art of wayfinding requires the wisdom of all Four Voices. Allow each voice to offer feedback and then, from the driver's seat of your life, determine your course of action.

### Name at least one small action step you can take to honor the feedback you've received.

Now it's time to take this inquiry practice off the page and into your life. Determine a small action step that you're willing to take to honor the feedback that you've received. Take a step in your new direction.

# Quick Review of the Four Voices Inquiry Method

1. What's one small thing you'd like to understand or get clear about?

2. What does your Mind Voice say about this?

3. What does your Heart Voice say about this?

4. What does your Body Voice say about this?

5. What does your Soul Voice say about this?

6. Specify your Point B for this particular situation.

7. Given the feedback of all Four Voices, what feels like the truest course of action for you to take at this time?

8. Name at least one small action step you can take to honor the feedback you've received.

*Example: Weekend Plans*

1. **What's one small thing you'd like to understand or get clear about?** I'm feeling pulled in a bunch of directions. Part of me wants to go away so that I'm not distracted. Part of me wants to have some alone time where no one asks me to do anything for them. Another part of me feels like I should stay home this weekend so that I can connect more deeply within my relationship. Simplifying this down to a question: Should I take some time to be alone this weekend, or should I stay home?

2. **What does your Mind Voice say about this?** Mind has a full-blown pity party. It's not fair that everyone else gets to have fun. It's not fair that I have to work this hard. I don't want to take care of anyone anymore. I need to be alone. I don't want to have to answer to anyone. I just want to go away and have my own bad mood. I don't want to connect right now. I want to disconnect. Interpretation: Mind wants to be alone.

3. **What does your Heart Voice say about this?** The most prevalent emotion is anger and frustration over having too many responsibilities. When I imagine being alone, I feel angry. When I imagine staying home to connect more deeply, I feel angry. It's not a clear read. Both options seem to have the feedback: Protect. I'm not sure what

I'm supposed to protect, but I'm interpreting this as: Heart wants to be alone.

4. **What does your Body Voice say about this?** When I imagine being alone, my body is tense and guarded. When I imagine connecting within my relationship, my body immediately relaxes. My body knows where it wants to be. It wants to be at home next to the person it trusts. Interpretation: Body wants to stay home and connect.

5. **What does your Soul Voice say about this?** When I check in with Soul, I get the answer: Both. Soul doesn't see this as an either/or problem. Soul wants to protect my sense of sovereignty and it wants to deeply connect within my relationship. I hadn't considered that I could do both until I checked in with Soul. Interpretation: Soul wants both.

6. **Specify your Point B for this particular situation.** I want to care for myself and for my intimate relationship. I want to live a life where I care for myself and for those around me.

7. **Given the feedback of all Four Voices, what feels like the truest course of action for you to take at this time?** Once I heard Soul's advice, it felt right to honor all Four Voices. Soul offered me the option of doing both. Rather than seeing this as a black and white question, I can see that the higher path is to connect deeply within my relationship by sharing what's really going on with me. This requires vulnerability, rather than isolation. This means that I ask for help with self-care, rather than just hiving myself away.

8. **Name at least one small action step you can take to honor the feedback you've received.** I will have an open and honest conversation about my inner frustrations and ask for help.

## Conclusion

# Point B

Your journey won't be a straight line. As you follow your Four Voices and begin living as your whole self, life itself will unfold in front of you. As you travel, new destinations and new roads will appear. Sometimes, you'll get close to Point B only to see that you'd rather go to Point C or Point D or Point E. Does that mean you won't get to Point B? Maybe. But that's not the point. Instead, it might mean you get close enough to see Point C. And when you get close to Point C, you might be able to see all the way to Point G.

When using all Four Voices, the very journey you travel transforms you. You become stronger, clearer, brighter. You no longer believe everything your mind says. You allow your heart to be wide open—trusting your inner emotions to give you direction. You no longer ignore the animal of your body—and you see it as a compassionate partner. Through this clarity, you're able to discern the subtle feedback from your soul.

Wayfinding with all Four Voices doesn't mean that they all agree. Often they won't. Rather, it means that each voice is heard and respected. Each voice has a job to do—it's up to you, the driver, to determine the direction you steer. It's up to you to determine which road to take. This is the work of your life: to stay awake, to keep your eyes open, to listen to all Four Voices, and to navigate life as your whole self.

And, no, sometimes you won't get to your original Point B, because the road you took to get there showed you broader horizons and greater destinations. With this new knowledge, you'll change your course and navigate in a new direction.

Whether you are on the mat or simply living your life, the art of wayfinding will open you to a sense of unity. Unity not only with your whole self, but unity with life itself. Connected to your whole self—grounding your mind in truth, living the full spectrum of your emotions, loving the animal of your body, and protecting the brilliance of your soul—you will find your own sense of vitality, inspiration, transformation, and healing. This union, this connection, this living from the driver's seat—this is yoga. No matter where you find yourself, how lost you feel, or how impossible your journey may seem, your Four Voices will always be there to guide you home.

Namaste.

# Resources

## Mind

For further study of the Mind Voice, I suggest:
*Loving What Is,* by Byron Katie
*The Power of Now,* by Eckhart Tolle

## Heart

For further study of the Heart Voice, I suggest:
*The Gifts of Imperfection: Let Go of Who You Think You're Supposed to Be and Embrace Who You Are,* by Brené Brown
*The Language of Emotions: What Your Feelings Are Trying to Tell You,* by Karla McKlaren
Yale University's course: *Human Emotion,* taught by Professor June Gruber (available on YouTube) for a greater understanding of evolutionary psychology.

## Body

For further study of the Body Voice, I suggest:
*Eastern Body, Western Mind* and *Wheels of Life*, both by Anodea Judith
*You Can Heal Your Life* and *Heal Your Body,* both by Louise Hay
*The Secret Language of Your Body,* by Inna Segal
*The Body Keeps the Score: Brain, Mind, and Body in the Healing of Trauma,* by Bessel van der Kolk, M.D.
*Healing Back Pain: The Mind-Body Connection,* by John E. Sarno

For shaking, I suggest music by Godfrey Mgcina, Nahini Doumbia, or the drumming compilation album *Drumming Planet.*

## Soul

For further study on the Soul Voice, I suggest:

*Inner Work: Using Dreams and Active Imagination for Personal Growth,* by
    Robert A. Johnson

*Joseph Campbell and The Power of Myth*, the 1988 PBS series hosted by Bill
    Moyers

The 1939 film *The Wizard of Oz*

My poetry suggestions include:

"Lost" by David Wagoner

"The Journey" by Mary Oliver

"Love After Love" by Derek Walcott

"House of Belonging" by David Whyte

"The Wild Iris" by Louise Glück

"Beannacht" by John O'Donohue

# Bibliography

Bell, Rob. "Episode 168: The One About Boundaries." *The Robcast.* Podcast audio October 15, 2017. https://robbell.podbean.com/e/the-one-about -boundaries/.

Campbell, Joseph. *Occidental Mythology.* New York: Penguin, 1991.

Gilbert, Elizabeth. *Eat, Pray, Love.* New York: Penguin Books, 2006.

Godden, Rumer. *A House with Four Rooms.* New York: William Morrow & Company, 1989.

Gruber, June. "Human Emotion 4.1: Evolution and Emotion, Yale University." Filmed May 2013. YouTube video, 21:14. Posted May 2013. https:// www.youtube.com/watch?v=fH-azxAhU-I.

Hemingway, Ernest. *A Moveable Feast.* New York: Charles Scribner's Sons, 1964.

Hillman, James. *The Soul's Code: In Search of Character and Calling.* New York: Random House, 1986.

Kondo, Marie, and Cathy Hirano. *The Life-changing Magic of Tidying Up: The Japanese Art of Decluttering and Organizing.* Berkeley: Ten Speed Press, 2014.

Sarno, John E. *Healing Back Pain: The Mind-Body Connection.* New York: Grand Central Publishing, 1991.

Satchidananda, Sri Swami. *The Yoga Sutra of Patanjali.* Virginia: Integral Yoga Publications, 1978.

Smith, Tiffany Watt. "The History of Human Emotions." Filmed November
    2017 at TED@Merck KGaA, Darmstadt, Germany, video 14:21, https://
    www.ted.com/talks/tiffany_watt_smith_the_history_of_human_emotions.

Taylor, Jill Bolte. *My Stroke of Insight: a Brain Scientist's Personal Journey.*
    New York: Viking, 2008.

Van der Kolk, Bessel A. *The Body Keeps the Score: Brain, Mind, and Body in
    the Healing of Trauma.* New York: Viking, 2014.

## To Write to the Author

If you wish to contact the author or would like more information about this book, please write to the author in care of Llewellyn Worldwide Ltd. and we will forward your request. Both the author and publisher appreciate hearing from you and learning of your enjoyment of this book and how it has helped you. Llewellyn Worldwide Ltd. cannot guarantee that every letter written to the author can be answered, but all will be forwarded. Please write to:

Meadow DeVor
℅ Llewellyn Worldwide
2143 Wooddale Drive
Woodbury, MN 55125-2989

Please enclose a self-addressed stamped envelope for reply,
or $1.00 to cover costs. If outside the U.S.A., enclose
an international postal reply coupon.

Many of Llewellyn's authors have websites with additional information and resources. For more information, please visit our website at http://www.llewellyn.com